When anorexia came to visit

Families talk about how an eating disorder invaded their lives

Bev Mattocks

CREATIVE
COPY

First published by Creative Copy 2013

www.creativecopy.co.uk

© Bev Mattocks 2013

Bev Mattocks asserts the moral right to be
identified as the author of this work

ISBN 978-0-9575118-4-2

IMPORTANT NOTE: This book contains true stories written from a personal
perspective. Each account is the sole expression and opinion of its contributors
and represents their own observations, memories, expression and recollections of
these events. Other people's opinions, observations, memories, expression and
recollections of the same events may differ. However, as far as the contributors can
recollect, allowing for the natural fallibility of memory, all the events depicted in
this book took place as described. To protect privacy, names have been changed.
The information provided in this book is not meant to be used, nor should it ever
be used, to diagnose or treat anorexia, bulimia, EDNOS or any other eating
disorder or medical condition. For diagnosis or treatment of anorexia, bulimia,
EDNOS or any other eating disorder or medical problem, please consult your own
physician. The writer and contributors do not endorse any specific eating disorder
treatment approach or model. Each individual is different and the strategies and
tips used and outlined in this book may not be suitable for other families. Also, any
references are provided for information purposes only and do not constitute
endorsement of any websites or other resources. Readers should also be aware that
the websites and other resources listed at the end of this book may change.

Find out more about Bev Mattocks at

www.anorexiaboy.co.uk

anorexiaboyrecovery.blogspot.co.uk

www.bevmattocks.co.uk

Contents

Dedication   i

About the author   ii

Foreword   iii
Professor Janet Treasure, OBE PhD FRCP FRCPsych, Director of the Eating Disorder Unit and Professor of Psychiatry at Kings College London

Preface   iv
Becky Henry, Founder & President of the Hope Network, LLC & Author of "Just Tell Her To Stop: Family Stories of Eating Disorders"

Introduction   viii
Laura Collins, Founder of F.E.A.S.T. & Author of "Eating With Your Anorexic"

About this book   xi
Bev Mattocks

Caroline's story   1
"When I look at Molly I want to show her to every desperate parent who has just discovered that their child has an eating disorder and say: 'This is what recovery looks like!'"

Marianne's story   15
"'Can you try and eat an apple?' the GP asked. I sat there open-mouthed. Lindy had almost stopped eating by this point. And, anyway, what difference would an extra 40 or 50 calories make?"

Vicky's story   23
"It's as if, all of a sudden, my daughter trusts us. She will now let me hug her. She'll talk, she'll chat and she's eating really well. Emotionally our 'little girl' is back with us again. It really is incredible."

Emma's story   32
"These days, she'll come in with a takeout, just like anyone else. She'll grab a burger here and a pizza there, or sit down in front of the telly with a tub of ice cream. She is just a really happy young lady."

Suzie's story   50
"I explained that we would never let her die, that we loved her and that she was too wonderful to lose. So whether we did it at home, in hospital or through a tube, we would ensure she got the nutrition she needed to get well."

Paul's & Jayne's story   60
"Eleanor took the information she picked up from appearing on Channel 4's Supersize vs Superskinny *and, by sheer willpower, applied it to herself. She refused to give in to the illness."*

Amanda's story   71
"'Just how far will you go?' I asked my daughter. 'There is no end,' she said. Terrified, I promised her there and then that, whether she hated me for the rest of her life, I was fighting for her very survival."

Gina's story   82
"I could see the consultant making notes, concluding that anxiety was the problem in the family and that our son was feeding off this atmosphere. Well of course we were anxious! What parents wouldn't be anxious?!"

Natalie's story   94
"The A&E nurse said: 'I'll go and get you a glass of squash; it won't be too much.' And there I was trying to explain that my daughter wouldn't even drink water, let alone squash."

Eva's story   102
"We parents know we have to get our children to eat. We know what they need to eat and how much of it they need to eat. The problem is, how do *we get them to eat?"*

Martha's story   111
"As a parent, I have not felt listened to during the whole of my daughter's illness. We may not be 'experts' but we still know our children best. And eating disorders appear to be one area of medicine where parental opinions are regularly ignored."

Tanya's story   117
"I remember going out to a restaurant and Lauren ordering a huge meal and a massive pudding with ice cream. It really was amazing, because she ate everything she was served up!"

Kathleen's story   128
"I can't tell you how desperate we were for someone to come and talk to us about the illness - to explain what we could expect, what was normal and what wasn't. We kept waiting. But there seemed to be nobody."

Elaine's story   143
"With someone like Lydia who doesn't handle change well, continuity is vital. But, at 18, patients are cut adrift from the treatment team they've come to know and trust to face the mysterious new world of Adult Services."

Dawn's story   153
"These days Karen will spend time with friends and will eat what they are eating. They'll have a pizza, even go across the road to the chip shop and have a deep fried Mars Bar. Who would have thought it?"

Heather's story   159
"While our child is being treated, we are busy learning too. And, unlike the professionals, we have no-one coaching us. All we have are books, internet sources and anyone else we can find whose brains are willing to be picked."

Adrienne's story   168
"I needed someone to hold my hand and tell me how to help my daughter but no-one seemed to have any answers. I felt totally helpless, isolated and very frightened. It was overwhelming."

Glenda's story   183
"Through the ATDT forum I realised that the re-feeding nightmare… the long periods sitting around the table, the awful atmosphere, the anger, the crying and all those things… were normal."

Sandra's story   192

"My son's anorexia helped me realise what is important in life. Many things seem so trivial compared to what we've been through. You see things in a different light. And that is good in a bizarre kind of way."

Shirley's story   198

"A teacher said: 'Here we are, talking about academic achievements. But, for Rebecca, walking into school every day is an achievement compared to these other students.' That was so lovely. Rebecca nearly cried. And so did I!"

Finally...   207

By the same author   212

Acknowledgements   215

Resources   217

Dedication

This book is dedicated to the wonderful families who have allowed me to share their stories with you in order that others might find inspiration and hope. It is also dedicated to the young people themselves, individuals who have demonstrated the courage, grit and sheer determination to fight this illness and win.

About the author

Bev Mattocks lives in the north of England with her husband and son, and works as a freelance advertising copywriter. She is a member of F.E.A.S.T. (Families Empowered And Supporting Treatment of Eating Disorders) and writes a popular blog about her experiences of supporting her teenage son through anorexia. She is the author of *Please Eat… A Mother's Struggle To Free Her Teenage Son From Anorexia* which is available from Amazon.

For more information, visit **www.anorexiaboy.co.uk**, **anorexiaboyrecovery.blogspot.co.uk** and **www.bevmattocks.co.uk**

Foreword

By Professor Janet Treasure, OBE PhD FRCP FRCPsych, Director of the Eating Disorder Unit and Professor of Psychiatry at Kings College London

When an eating disorder comes to visit, friends and families are often the first to know. Furthermore families can play a key role in mentoring the process of recovery and moderating the isolation that causes the illness to become stuck.

However this illness is not like other illnesses. It pervades all aspects of family life. Additionally, a starved brain results in the individual being less able to manage the skills required for successful inter-personal processes. A vicious circle starts. As a result, family members need high levels of emotional intelligence and practical skills to interrupt this downward spiral and guide their child towards recovery.

When Anorexia Came To Visit: Families Talk About How An Eating Disorder Invaded Their Lives details the recovery stories of 20 individuals from the family perspective. These stories offer hope and resilience through their honesty and practical advice and will be an invaluable source of support for families.

Professor Janet Treasure, OBE PhD FRCP FRCPsych

Preface

By Becky Henry, Founder & President of the Hope Network, LLC & Award Winning Author of "Just Tell Her To Stop: Family Stories of Eating Disorders"

Myths and misconceptions about the nature and causes of eating disorders are still endemic. Thankfully, understanding of these complex and life-threatening illnesses is increasing as new and more effective evidence-based treatments are being developed. Across the world, enlightened healthcare professionals are coming to realise that a collaborative approach between professionals and families can result in a better outcome for the patient. As a professional certified coach, a Board Member of F.E.A.S.T. (Families Empowered And Supporting Treatment of Eating Disorders) and a parent that actively advocates for evidence-based treatment through my organization the *Hope Network* in the USA, I look forward to the day when all healthcare professionals will recognise the urgent need to update their understanding, treatment and care of people with eating disorders.

During the two years between 2000 and 2002, while I was failing to get my daughter's eating disorder diagnosed, I had no idea that parents across the world were struggling with similar problems.

After taking my daughter to the pediatrician and two psychologists over those two years, the long path to treatment came only after I handed the pediatrician the diagnosis on a silver platter - my daughter's friends had finally shared with me the frightening details of what was going on. I gave the pediatrician this evidence and insisted on a referral. Unfortunately, back then, the local eating disorders treatment center was still practicing the old "parentectomy" model where we, as parents, were asked to "back off" and leave it to the health professionals to care for our daughter. As a result her eating disorder was permitted to distort her perceptions of what was being said and done and we were not included to counter this. I wish I'd been armed with these words from *A Collaborative Approach to Eating Disorders* (edited by June Alexander & Professor Janet Treasure OBE, PhD FRCP FRCPsych, Director of the Eating Disorder Unit and Professor of Psychiatry at Kings College London): "Families are now seen as integral to the treatment of children and adolescents with eating disorders... Family-based treatment has been shown to be effective in the treatment of adolescent AN [Anorexia Nervosa]."

During my struggles with my daughter's eating disorder I searched for connection with other parents and for more information about effective treatments. This difficult and isolating experience is what drove me to interview over 40 families and write their stories for my book *Just Tell Her To Stop: Family Stories Of Eating Disorders* (published in January 2011) so that other families would have information and feel less isolated.

I have also made it my mission as Founder & President of the *Hope Network* to share information on evidence-based treatment with healthcare providers in order that patients can be diagnosed and treated sooner. Eating disorders are like any other serious illness in that earlier intervention is more effective than waiting until it is entrenched.

As with other mental health illnesses over the decades, it can take multiple sources singing the same tune to change entrenched and redundant theories. I'll never forget being at a conference on eating disorders in the United States in September 2010. Princeton University had sponsored Dr Walter Kaye (Director of the Eating Disorders Program, Professor, University of California San Diego Department of Psychiatry) and Professor Janet Treasure OBE

(Director of the Eating Disorder Unit and Professor of Psychiatry at Kings College London) to teach us about the neuroscience of eating disorders.

After listening to a three-hour explanation about the intricacies of the brain's role in eating disorders, I was thrilled to have scientific evidence disproving the lingering, outdated belief that poor parenting causes eating disorders. So you can imagine my dismay when, over lunch, a psychotherapist who had been working in the field for many years leaned over to me and said: "There may be some truth in what these two are saying but if it weren't for pathological parents, we wouldn't have eating disorders."

Thankfully, Dr Kaye, Professor Treasure and others are pioneers in spreading the message that eating disorders are biological brain illnesses and that parents are part of the solution, not the problem.

I am very grateful for all the wonderful reviews and feedback on my book *Just Tell Her To Stop* from both families and healthcare providers in and outside of the USA. As these are such complex and prevalent disorders, we need many, many similar stories to help people understand and let go of outdated information.

It was with great joy that I learned about June Alexander's book, *My Kid Is Back: Empowering Parents to Beat Anorexia Nervosa* (February 2010) which shares stories of families in Australia fighting eating disorders using FBT (Family-Based Treatment). And now I am thrilled to hear of Bev Mattocks' latest book *When Anorexia Came To Visit* which shares the stories of 20 families in the UK who have undergone, and in some cases are still undergoing, treatment.

Of course diagnosis can be complex. As I said in my book *Just Tell Her To Stop*, as much as we would wish it to be so, there is no one-size-fits-all treatment and what is important is to find the right treatment for your child. Bev Mattocks' book - like mine - is not meant to endorse any particular treatment model; merely to let you know what is available. It is not a medical reference; it is a book of real stories describing different circumstances and treatment approaches.

As with my book, Bev has gathered together these stories because she, and the book's contributors, do not want other families to go through the same nightmare. The families described in this book want to offer hope to others by showing what worked (and what was less successful) in their individual circumstances. I hope that other families may be able to draw inspiration from these accounts and feel empowered when approaching their treatment providers.

The other purpose of Bev's book is to show healthcare professionals what goes on at home, beyond the confines of the consulting room. And, as parents who are living with this illness on the front line for many, many exhausting hours a week, I look forward to the day when it will be accepted practice for parents to be recognised as a vital part of the treatment team.

Within the pages of *When Anorexia Came To Visit* you will read many positive and inspirational stories of hope - of excellent GPs and healthcare professionals working with parents to get the child well. But you will also read stories where families have battled with, and in some cases are still battling with, inadequate services and treatment, especially evident once a child reaches the age of 18 and no longer qualifies for adolescent services.

I hope that, with multiple books like this one, the tide will shift and outdated theories will finally be put to rest - and that funds will be spent on ensuring people have access to high quality treatment wherever they live. It is thanks to pioneers like Bev Mattocks, June Alexander and others that these stories are being told which will, I hope, help to turn this tide and get these most deadly of all mental illnesses the research, recognition and understanding that is needed.

Becky Henry, Founder & President of the Hope Network,
LLC & Award Winning Author of "Just Tell Her To Stop:
Family Stories of Eating Disorders"

Introduction

Laura Collins, Founder of F.E.A.S.T. (Families Empowered And Supporting Treatment of Eating Disorders) & Author of "Eating With Your Anorexic" explains about the F.E.A.S.T. community and its online forum Around The Dinner Table (ATDT)

I hear lots of questions when a parent realizes their child has an eating disorder. The question that comes up most often is: "Where can I find other families who have survived this?"

Before the diagnosis, few of us will have talked with another family facing anorexia, bulimia or another eating disorder. So when we discover our child is sick, we can feel alone, isolated and frightened. We want to know that there is hope; that our child will recover - and we want to meet other parents that have faced the crisis and come out the other side. Indeed talking to families that have survived an eating disorder can be one of the most encouraging and empowering comforts during difficult times.

Bev Mattocks has collected together just some of these stories, many from a very special place: the Around The Dinner Table forum - an online forum run by parents *for* parents. ATDT (as it is often known) began in late 2004 with only one member: me. I started it because I envisioned a community of parents helping other parents to survive this devastating experience. I knew that the internet was an ideal place because it's low-cost, open 24 hours, international and anonymous. When a mother or father is desperately searching for information and inspiration the ATDT forum is like a lighthouse on a stormy night, showing the way to safety. What started out with me asking my relatives and friends to "please post something" is now a longstanding institution with thousands of families that have come to us for support.

The generosity of the community that developed at ATDT continues to amaze me. There are caring folks there at all hours to offer leads to information, provide inspiration or simply a friendly shoulder to cry on during stressful moments. These fathers and mothers give willingly of their experience and show genuine compassion for one another. The number of readers always exceeds the ones writing so we know that the experiences of our users have a wider impact and will continue to do so for years.

ATDT is run by a wonderful group of volunteers. The moderator team - or "Mod Squad" - know our vast archives inside out and can refer a new parent to relevant "threads" whether current or past. British, Canadian, American, New Zealand or Australian families find one another, families facing similar symptoms find one another, and those living near enough to actually meet for coffee form invaluable local support networks across the globe.

By using the power of the internet, even with its drawbacks, ATDT has been able to offer support that is found nowhere else. Many practicing clinicians tell us they learned of a new technique, book or other information source from reading the forum. I regularly hear from parents that ATDT was an essential tool in their family's success. Indeed many of the families in *When Anorexia Came To Visit* describe ATDT as a "lifesaver" during the darkest days.

Because we are a peer-to-peer environment, one of our rules is that we are limited to our own experiences. We do not tell other parents what to do or how to think. We share our stories so that others can use our experiences in making their own decisions. This isn't always easy: at times every one of us wants to say, "You should..."

The limitation of an online forum, however, is that each story is told in individual "threads" over time. Rarely can you follow a family's whole story through one "thread." This is what makes a book like *When Anorexia Came To Visit* so important. I applaud Bev Mattocks for gathering these stories and giving these 20 wonderful families a voice.

Of course with such a complex illness and widely differing personal circumstances, every story is different. Nonetheless there will be overlaps and elements that families will recognise and identify with. Like me and countless others, you will read these stories and find yourself nodding your head and saying "Me, too!" as you hear about families undergoing similar experiences to your own.

May these stories, and these brave families, offer you the hope and inspiration you need and deserve in the fight for full and sustained recovery. Your story, too, is yet to be told!

Laura Collins, Founder of F.E.A.S.T.
& Author of "Eating With Your Anorexic"

About this book

By Bev Mattocks

One thing I remember saying over and over again to my husband - and probably still say on occasions - is this: "We should have picked up on it sooner."

The question is: could we, or any of the families I interviewed for this book, have "picked up on our child's eating disorder sooner"?

When I first took my 15-year old son, Ben, to visit the GP at the end of September 2009, the signs of an emerging eating disorder had been evident for some months.

The problem was that we didn't recognise them.

Even before the signs emerged, the eating disorder was busy germinating in the inner recesses of Ben's mind. He says he can trace it back to at least 12 months before, if not earlier.

The fact is that you don't expect your child to develop an eating disorder. You don't expect it to happen to your ordinary, happy, close family. And, in our case, and a couple of other cases in this book, you don't expect it to happen to your son.

Eating disorders aren't like "normal" medical conditions where recognisable symptoms are there for all to see: a broken bone, a worrying lump, blood loss or whatever - the kind of issues that GPs deal with on a daily basis. And, although eating disorders often feature in the media, they rarely focus on the lesser known signs and symptoms, preferring instead to major on shock tactics such as stereotypical skeletal photographs. On top of this there is the popular misconception that eating disorders are "caused" by anything from bad parenting and size zero fashion models to faddy eaters and even private schooling (how many reports begin with: *"Privately educated XXXX...."*?)

So, during the early months as the illness began to manifest itself, few of the families in *When Anorexia Came To Visit* had any idea what they were dealing with. Nor did their children. For instance it's not as if my son sat down one day and decided to "get anorexia". He was as ignorant as any of us. And, anyway, these days we know that anorexia is a biologically-based mental illness, not a lifestyle choice.

But we didn't know this back then.

Indeed none of the families in this book fits the stereotype of the dysfunctional family with the child who is going off the rails and chooses, perhaps as a "control thing", to starve themselves to death. Before anorexia came to visit they were just ordinary happy families living ordinary happy lives. And our children were *normal*.

So there was no reason on this planet why any of us would have been watching out for the classic signs of anorexia. This is why we couldn't have "picked up on it sooner" unless we'd known what to look out for.

None of us knew that a whole package of horrors comes with an eating disorder. It's not just about cutting back on food and losing weight, it's about crushing depression, vicious mood swings, violent self-harming, suicide threats and social isolation as your child transforms into someone you don't recognise, right in front of your eyes. Our son even developed a different voice: a slow, low, deep monotone that used to chill me to the core.

We weren't aware that an eating disorder creeps up on its victim ever so slowly, so slowly that it's almost undetectable until it's got a firm hold. We didn't know that, in the early months, an eating disorder can disguise itself as a passion for healthy eating and / or exercise, or a passion for cooking. Or, in the case of our son Ben, all three.

None of us knew of the devastating effect that anorexia would have on the whole family - from the sufferer themselves through to siblings, parents, grandparents and the extended family. Not just for a brief few weeks or months, but sometimes for years.

And we didn't know that you don't always have to be a skin-and-bones skeleton to have full-blown anorexia.

But, despite our obliviousness to the early signs, most of the families I interviewed for this book expressed feelings of intense guilt. "Why didn't we notice what was happening?", "Why didn't we act sooner?" and "Why didn't we trust our gut instincts that something was wrong?"

And here lies another problem. All too often, healthcare professionals are also failing to recognise the clear warning signs of an eating disorder and take appropriate action urgently.

In the making of this book I talked to GPs, medical students, even the Royal College of General Practitioners (RCGP), and there seems to be very little formal training in eating disorders in the UK. Our local GP said she "probably had two lectures" as a medical student at Cambridge. A medical student specialising in psychiatry appeared surprised to learn from my family that males get eating disorders. And a representative from the RCGP told me that: "Currently only around 50 per cent of doctors-in-training for general practice have an opportunity to undertake specialist-led mental health or in child health training placements (e.g. based in hospitals or specialist mental health services) during their three-year GP training programme." (However I understand that proposals are in place for this to change.)

The fact is that, when you take your child to the GP, you expect them to know what is wrong and take action. So, when a GP fails to identify an eating disorder or assumes it's "just a teenage phase", you begin to doubt your own instincts. After all, they're the professionals, they should know.

And, meanwhile, your child can be in complete denial that there is anything wrong. So sometimes it can be just you, the parent, puzzling over whether or not you should be worried - and then fighting a lone battle to get your child diagnosed and referred.

Thankfully, once referred, most of the families in this book saw a service like CAMHS (Child & Adolescent Mental Health Services) very quickly, sometimes within the week. Out of all the families in this book I think we had to wait the longest. It was four months from our first GP visit before we saw our local CAMHS team and only then because the assessment was expedited when Ben's pulse plummeted to 29 and he ended up wired up to machines in hospital.

Just because your child has been referred, it doesn't automatically mean they are going to receive exemplary, informed, evidence-based treatment. From my discussions with families, whether or not your child receives effective treatment appears to vary according to where you live. Additionally, some children are being referred to generalised mental health services like CAMHS whereas others are being referred to specialist eating disorders centres. In areas where there is very little available, or where a child's BMI is not considered "low enough" to qualify for treatment, families are being forced to opt for costly private care. Sometimes the NHS agrees to pay for this private treatment and sometimes it doesn't. Sometimes children are admitted into an eating disorders unit as inpatients and sometimes treatment providers prefer to keep them as outpatients. To us, as "lay" parents, there doesn't seem to be any consistent pattern, and this comes across clearly in the large cross-section of families I spoke to in the making of this book and on many other occasions - families from across the UK, including Scotland and Wales.

One of the many reasons why I decided to write this book is because I wanted to see how our own personal story (described in my book *Please Eat... A Mother's Struggle To Free Her Teenage Son From Anorexia*) overlaps with other families' experiences across the UK.

Of course each family's circumstances are different. Yet so much of what we've experienced is similar. Not just in terms of the warning signs but in the way the illness transformed our children into people we scarcely recognised, mentally as well as physically. And, of course, the sheer uphill struggle of trying to get them to eat again.

In this book you will read some truly uplifting accounts: those stories where intervention was swift and the illness was tackled by a coordinated team of clinicians using the latest evidence-based treatment focusing on full nutrition first and foremost, and recognising parents as an integral part of the recovery process.

But you will also read about families who experienced the other end of the spectrum - those mental health services that "could do better". With these families recovery didn't come as quickly; some are still a work in progress.

I often wonder where parents would be without the power of the internet. Would we still be ignorant of the latest evidence-based treatment? Would we still accept the outdated notion that eating disorders have to last for several years, if not for life? Would we still believe that eating disorders "aren't really about food" and are "a control thing"? Would we still be dragging our children to dozens of pointless sessions as therapists attempt to identify the "reasons why" the eating disorder developed and talk them out of the illness? Would close family relationships have disintegrated as parents, wrongly labelled at best as dysfunctional and at worst as abusive, needlessly blame each other for "causing" the illness?

There is an online resource called F.E.A.S.T. (Families Empowered And Supporting Treatment of Eating Disorders), set up by Laura Collins, author of *Eating With Your Anorexic* (who was kind enough to write the Introduction for this book). F.E.A.S.T. and its online forum, Around The Dinner Table (ATDT), is run by parents and carers *for* parents and carers. Today F.E.A.S.T. is widely respected by some of the world's leading eating disorder professionals and its website is a mine of information on the latest evidence-based treatment, research and resources. Thanks to F.E.A.S.T. and other resources such as the UK eating disorder charities Beat and ABC (Anorexia & Bulimia Care) families can educate themselves about the latest advances in the treatment of eating disorders in a way that was previously impossible.

The ATDT forum is a place where families can come and feel immediately welcome, among families who understand exactly what they are going through and who can offer support. Here in the UK we have established a truly awesome network that works with other charities like Beat and leading eating disorder experts to advocate better treatment for our children and enhanced support for parents and carers.

Virtually every family in this book says that F.E.A.S.T. and ATDT were lifesavers. It is also thanks to the people I've met through F.E.A.S.T. and Beat that I have been able to gather together these 20 powerful, insightful and inspiring stories.

Through this book, we want to show other families that they are not to blame for their child's illness. Eating disorders are biologically-based mental illnesses, not lifestyle choices. And, yes, eating disorders *are* about food - lots of it, being administered by strong, loving, dedicated families who refuse to accept that their beloved child is "in this for the long haul". We know that you can't "talk someone out of an eating disorder"; you can't wait for someone to "want to get better". And we recognise that parents are a vital part of a successful, highly coordinated treatment team. We parents are part of the solution, not the problem.

We also want to show other families what is "normal" in the world of eating disorder behaviour. Distressing and terrifying, yes, but relatively "normal" for a child in the iron grip of anorexia. And also what is normal as the brain begins to get re-nourished, gradually heals and returns to its pre-anorexia state.

Finally, we want to show that, no matter what you are going through, other families have been through it too and successfully come out the other side - and the tools and coping strategies that we found most helpful.

What this book isn't, however, is a medical reference. It is not meant to be used, nor should it ever be used, to diagnose or treat an eating disorder. For diagnosis or treatment you should always consult your own physician. Nor does this book endorse any particular treatment model or approach, or any particular eating disorders clinic, hospital, unit or treatment provider. Eating disorders are notoriously complex and diverse illnesses, and a one-size-fits-all approach to treatment is nigh impossible. In other words, everything contained within the pages of this book is for information purposes only including the tips at the end of chapters which are based on individual experiences. In other words, what worked for one family may be inappropriate for another so please be sure to consult your physician or eating disorders specialist. Also, to protect privacy, names have been changed and locations have been disguised.

Additionally, I would suggest keeping this book away from your child. As Becky Henry says in the Introduction to her book *Just Tell Her To Stop: Family Stories Of Eating Disorders*, there may be statements that could be "triggering" to the eating disorder. Becky says: "The stories in the book could 'teach the eating disorder' new tricks to further compromise your loved one's health." For this reason, in *When Anorexia Came To Visit*, I have taken care to remove references to, or disguise, specific "tricks". However some things need to be shared in order that parents can be aware that these things happen and remain vigilant.

Getting your child through an eating disorder is one of the toughest and most distressing things you will ever do as a parent. But re-visiting painful memories is unbelievably tough, too. Yet each of the families I interviewed for this book willingly volunteered to come forward and describe their own struggles with anorexia.

Not only did they agree to talk frankly about their experiences, they agreed to read through the various drafts I sent through for checking. In other words, being involved in this book meant having to re-visit distressing memories not once but several times over. This takes courage and commitment. It also demonstrates how much these families care about others - families they have never met who will read this book and hopefully draw inspiration, strength and hope from its pages.

This book could never have been written without the help of these 20 fantastic families. In many cases all I have done, as the author, is to edit the transcript of a taped conversation or tweak a detailed written account. So, strictly, I should be calling myself *editor*, not *author*. These 20 families and the three wonderful people who provided the *Foreword, Preface* and *Introduction* have written this book, not me. And I am immensely appreciative of their help, dedication and input.

Finally I must thank the young people themselves for demonstrating the courage, grit and determination to fight the eating disorder and win. Being a parent is tough, but being someone who has fought to break free from this insidious illness is even tougher.

Our sons and daughters are truly awesome.

And so are their parents.

Bev Mattocks, July 2013

When anorexia came to visit

Families talk about how an eating disorder invaded their lives

Caroline's story

"When I look at Molly I want to show her to every desperate parent who has just discovered that their child has an eating disorder and say: 'This is what recovery looks like!'"

You don't expect your normal, level-headed, beautiful and intelligent daughter to get anorexia. Like many people I assumed that eating disorders happened to other families. I assumed they were "caused" by traumatic events, being brought up in a dysfunctional family environment, the pressure in the media to be stick thin or a whole range of other "causes" that weren't relevant to our close, happy, normal family.

So when our university student daughter, Molly, began to show signs of an eating disorder, my first reaction was shock. How could this happen to us? My second was the realisation that I knew *nothing* about this illness that seemed to be consuming my daughter. Yes, I'd read sensational stories in newspapers and magazines and I knew of a couple of girls at Molly's old school who'd developed eating disorders, but apart from that I knew nothing.

Molly was in her second year at university in Cambridge. She'd come home for the Christmas holidays and from the moment she arrived through the front door it was clear that something was wrong. She was edgy, irritable and demanding. Molly and I had planned a night at the ballet; it was a favourite annual ritual. We'd have dinner at a favourite restaurant and then go onto the theatre. It was a real mother and daughter treat and we looked forward to it

1

immensely. Over dinner Molly was unusually difficult and refused to have a dessert. In the past desserts had always been a favourite. I wasn't big on home cooking, but apple pies and crumbles from Marks & Spencer were always firm favourites. But on this occasion, Molly refused to share even a small dessert.

Molly didn't speak to me in the cab we shared to Sadlers Wells. It was as if she were cross with me; as if I'd done something wrong. At the theatre I went to the bar to get a drink and when I returned I was shocked to find her sobbing in a corner. When I tried to comfort her, she told me that she was hearing "voices" in her head. She said they were telling her she shouldn't like me because I was trying to make her fat. My first reaction was shock closely followed by an intense fear as it suddenly dawned on me that something was seriously wrong.

The ballet was Cinderella. But I don't remember much about the performance. Every now and again I glanced across at Molly and she seemed absorbed in the action on the stage as though the bombshell she had just dropped had never happened. We drove home afterwards and made polite conversation about anything except the thing we most needed to talk about. Back home, Molly thanked me for a "lovely evening" and went to bed. I numbly recounted the evening to my husband, Graham, who seemed very calm about the whole thing and suggested this was maybe something many teenagers went through.

Suddenly, over the next few days, I began to notice everything I should have noticed before. Molly was extremely anxious. She was constantly cold and I became aware of a soft downy sort of hair on her face which wasn't there before. Molly was also exercising more. She'd always been interested in sport, but really only as a spectator. She was the type of child who would come last in most of the races, but would always cross the line with a huge smile on her face, glad to have been a competitor, but never competitive. But now she was swimming 100 lengths of the pool, and running most days and in all weathers. I couldn't help noticing that she didn't seem to be getting any enjoyment out of it. Whatever the weather, she'd be out there, often carrying injuries to her ankles or shins, but driven to run regardless.

I also noticed that Molly was drinking huge amounts of water and cutting food into small pieces. Hot drinks were always black coffee and these days she never had milk. Oddly she had no problem eating fruit, but she wouldn't drink a glass of fruit juice. Requests for her to eat were met with the same responses: "I've already eaten", "I'm not hungry" or "I'll eat later".

My first reaction was guilt. Why hadn't I noticed before? Over Christmas I watched her with new eyes and started to see how anxious and unhappy she seemed. Hanging her clothes on the line after washing them, I was struck by how small her jeans were and realised that my next door neighbour's daughter's clothes looked to be about the same size, and she wasn't even 10 years old.

I frantically wanted to "fix" things, but I didn't know what to do. Oh, and I was angry with Graham who didn't seem to be as frightened as I was. Graham has always been very calm and undramatic. I didn't seem to be able to make him understand that I thought we had a really big problem on our hands.

Our GP seemed to be the first port of call. Molly agreed she needed to go because, fundamentally, she's a pleaser and she could see how worried I was. To be honest, I think she felt very ambivalent about me at this time. Part of her wanted to make me happy. But the other part of her believed I was either the problem or I had *caused* the problem. At this stage no-one had mentioned the words "eating disorder" let alone "anorexia" and in my head I still didn't put the two things together. I was absolutely in denial about what was happening. It was almost as if by giving it a name it would suddenly become real.

That first visit to the local GP left me feeling very discouraged. I had checked online to see which of the six GPs in our practice had experience of eating disorders. Naïvely I thought there would be someone that specialised in the illness. But, instead, I had to settle for a GP who had a special interest in mental health issues.

The GP weighed Molly and agreed she was underweight. She also suggested we see a therapist to help her with her attitude to food and come back for a fortnightly weigh-in at the surgery. But I explained that it wouldn't be possible because Molly was away at university. So we agreed that Molly would visit her GP in Cambridge to seek help.

I remember feeling uneasy. Although the GP specialised in mental health, she admitted to us that she knew nothing about eating disorders. To her credit, though, she said she was willing to learn. But the thing is, when you take your child to see the GP you expect them to know what is wrong and how to deal with it. I felt as if she knew as little as me. So I hoped and prayed that the university GP would be able to help.

So, Molly returned to Cambridge where she saw one of the university's GPs. After a full psychological assessment, she was diagnosed with restrictive anorexia nervosa. I wasn't with her the day she was diagnosed, and I still hate myself for not being there. I know from talking to Molly later that the visit left her frightened and confused. The GP suggested that Molly saw a CBT therapist (Cognitive Behavioural Therapy) for help with her "issues", so I found a private therapist in Cambridge and Molly started to see her once a week. During this time she continued to lose weight steadily

It was four months before Molly was finally referred for specialist eating disorders treatment during which time she continued to lose weight. Every time I went to university to visit her or she came home she seemed to be thinner. By the time she was referred her weight was very low indeed. In fact, in my opinion, Molly was critical by this stage.

The days were punctuated with constant phone calls from Molly - always in tears, often frightened because she was trying to face the traumas presented by eating a biscuit, or more often, *not* eating a biscuit. I dreaded my phone ringing because I knew she would always be in distress. She'd complain of feeling constantly cold and permanently tired. When Graham and I visited, we dreaded leaving her, knowing she would be crying and so very miserable with her life.

I spent hours on the computer researching anything and everything to do with eating disorders. There was just so much to learn! I thought: "Where on earth do I start?" I knew absolutely nothing about eating disorders.

Then, one day, I came across a website from a charity called F.E.A.S.T. I made contact with Laura Collins, F.E.A.S.T.'s founder in the States, who was a mine of information. I was surprised that Laura responded personally to my first desperate email. I must have sounded like a half-crazed mad woman; asking lots of questions and needing lots of answers. Laura responded calmly and with huge empathy, reassuring me that there was a way to beat the illness and encouraging me to stay calm and take control.

She gave me a reading list. I devoured *Help Your Teenager Beat an Eating Disorder* by David Lock & Daniel Le Grange and *Skills-Based Learning For Caring For A Loved One With An Eating Disorder: The New Maudsley Method* by Janet Treasure. On top of this I was on the internet every night, more often than not on F.E.A.S.T.'s online forum: Around The Dinner Table. I tortured myself reading first-hand accounts of other parents describing the hell they were going through as they sought to save their children from various manifestations of eating disorders. I was in turn comforted and reassured by all the resources on the F.E.A.S.T. website including links to academic papers that confirmed the biological nature of the illness. This was where I learned that we, as parents, didn't *cause* the eating disorder. Neither did our daughter *choose* to develop anorexia. Eating disorders are not a lifestyle choice; they are biological brain disorders in the same way that a whole range of mental health illnesses are brain disorders.

I was worried about the fact that, as a legal adult, I might be excluded from Molly's treatment. By then I'd learned enough to know that, in theory, I had the right to choose where I wanted her to receive help and I thought we would agree to a referral to the local eating disorders unit to see if it was any good. If it wasn't, then I assumed we could ask for a referral to another hospital. Our GP had recommended one particular hospital, but on closer investigation I discovered they didn't have a unit for adults with eating disorders, only children.

I had real reservations about our local eating disorders unit. Their website was shocking. It mentioned about 12 different types of talking therapies as treatment for anorexia. To me this seemed odd because, although we were looking at an eating disorders unit, nowhere on the website was there any mention of food or the importance of early intervention and restoring the patient to a healthy weight. From what I could see the idea seemed to be that you could *talk* the patient out of the eating disorder.

Within a month of being referred, Molly was sitting in front of the consultant who headed up the eating disorders unit at the local hospital, and a CBT therapist. I felt an almost instant antipathy with the consultant who conducted that first meeting with Molly without me present. He made lots of reassuring noises but maintained that Molly needed to sort out her underlying issues before she could start to eat again

In the event the treatment was pretty worthless. Molly attended around 30 CBT sessions which she said were useless. She'd sit in a warm, darkened room with a very nice lady who explored her relationships with her step-siblings and parents. How, I often wondered, was all this probing and talking supposed to help my daughter to recover from this devastating illness?

In my conversations with the consultant he gave me every indication that he thought I was an archetypal control freak. I hated myself for appearing to be so controlling. But the fact is that I wanted answers and I wanted them quickly. I didn't want to hear that "you're in this for the long haul", "the average length of time for recovery is between five and seven years" or "this may be something she never really recovers from". I refused to let this be the prognosis for my much-loved daughter and doubtless this is why I may have appeared to be "controlling".

The eating disorders unit seemed to have a culture of resignation and I wanted us to be the ones that proved it wrong. The consultant thought I was naïve; I thought he needed to educate himself about the latest evidence-based treatment for eating disorders. During one conversation I mentioned the Minnesota Experiment (a clinical study at the University of Minnesota in the 1940s to determine the physiological and psychological effects of severe and prolonged dietary restriction and the effectiveness of dietary rehabilitation strategies). The consultant smiled patronisingly and said: "Well, why am I not surprised that you've read about that?!"

Then all of a sudden we had another trauma to deal with. Within weeks of Molly's treatment, my husband Graham suffered a massive heart attack and was rushed into Harefield Hospital for open heart surgery. He was there for three weeks, during which time Molly took leave from university. Those three weeks were the worst of my life. Molly seemed like a stranger. On the day of her father's open heart surgery, she refused to come with me to visit him in Intensive Care, saying she was going for a run instead. I knew this was her way of dealing with her own stress and incredible guilt (I later found out that she believed she had caused his heart attack), but it was so uncharacteristic of her. It showed just how much the illness had changed her. My lovely girl had gone and had been replaced with a selfish, self-obsessed stranger.

When Graham came home from hospital, Molly returned to university. But within the week she was back home again. A member of F.E.A.S.T. who just happened to be her Russian tutor had asked Molly to get me to call her. This tutor had experience of dealing with anorexia as her own daughter had struggled with the illness several years before and made a full recovery.

That phone call changed everything. It empowered me to take control and stop feeling so helpless. After all, I had two people to look after now. I decided not to wait for anyone else to help us, believing that the best way to get Molly well was to feed her back to health. I wasn't sure at that time if just restoring her to a healthy

7

weight would be sufficient, but I knew enough by then to know that nothing else was likely to improve until this happened.

Getting Molly to eat was going to be a hard fought battle and I needed to devote myself to it full-time. I quit my job the following day, drove to get Molly and battened down the hatches for the months to come. Luckily my job offered me a six month sabbatical to nurse Graham and Molly. We took out a bank loan to cover my lost salary for this period and, with the support of the ATDT forum and what I had learned through reading and so on, we began to re-feed Molly at home. We agreed that Molly would return to Cambridge to take her second year exams and the rest of the time she would remain at home. We left her lovely long standing boyfriend in Cambridge, with his full support and agreement that this was the best chance we had of getting Molly well.

It took seven months to get Molly back to a healthy weight - the hardest seven months of my life. In that time we treated every week as a challenge to gain at least a pound in weight. The routine was always the same. Breakfast at 8am, morning coffee and cake at 10.30am, lunch at 1pm, and dinner at 7pm. I prepared all the meals, plated them and served them - and always ate exactly the same as Molly. Sometimes meals went smoothly and sometimes they didn't.

There were some horrendous scenes, with food thrown in the bin and meals having to be cooked all over again. Sometimes Molly left the house and I was terrified that she wouldn't return. There were screaming rages and scenes in the street. I can't really describe how awful it was.

There were two occasions when I went to bed and prayed I wouldn't wake up - anything to end it all and make it go away. It was a while before I learned that my distress only fuelled Molly's anxiety and made her worse. I had to learn to stay calm and become the world's greatest actress. Nothing was an issue, everything was fine, I was so R-E-L-A-X-E-D and we were going to get through this.

Sixteen months on Molly remains at a healthy weight yet still struggles daily with the remnants of her illness. She eats well and enjoys her food and my beautiful girl is back. She is changed by what she has been through and I am so proud of her. She describes her illness as an "evil voice" in her head, but understands now that this was something she was probably born with - a genetic predisposition towards an eating disorder and that, somewhere along the way, a failure to match the necessary intake of food with the growing she was doing in her adolescence tipped her into anorexia.

The difference is that, these days, Molly recognises the illness for what it is. She never wants to get sick again and knows what she needs to do to stay well. Indeed she's told me how terrified she is of the anorexia coming back and I believe it's this fear that keeps her eating. When she's stressed, for example when studying becomes too much, I can almost see it creep up on her, like an Achilles heel that the eating disorder takes advantage of. Often I have to sit down with her and point out all the positives, talk to her about the future she deserves to have, the family she deserves to have, and all the little things that have changed in order to show her just how far she has come.

Molly is bright and sensitive. She gets it. She knows she has been to hell and back and never wants to go there again. She says she feels embarrassed now when she thinks about how she behaved when she was so sick, so she tries not to think about it. I tell her it wasn't really her. That person was the one who had been hijacked by anorexia. Molly was buried in there all the time, desperate to get out.

Molly returned to university in September 2012 after a gap of 17 months. Graham or I visit her at least once a week for a meal. We talk openly to her about managing the risks that the illness exposes her to. We agree that it would not be wise for her to resume exercising again. She does a lot of walking and enjoys cycling with her boyfriend, but solitary running and swimming would not be good for her. She understands that she needs to make time for herself and have a good balance between work and play. It has been a joy in the last six months to hear her recount stories of dances she has been to, having one glass of wine too many, buying a new dress in an acceptable size - all normal student things.

Going back to those early months it's clear that our GP had limited awareness of eating disorders. I felt as if I knew more about the illness than she did, and, at the time, my own knowledge was pretty patchy. But, once I'd done the research, I actually felt I knew more about the latest evidence-based approaches than the consultant at the eating disorder unit. The health professionals we interacted with throughout Molly's illness all seemed to share the same view that Molly had an eating disorder that needed intensive psychological therapy, and this was best accomplished with Molly on her own.

I remember being reduced to tears on several occasions.

On one occasion when Molly was being interviewed while I sat in the waiting room outside, the therapist asked her why she felt *I wanted her to gain weight*. Molly replied that she thought it was because I wanted her to get well. His response was: "What *other* reason do you think your mother could have for wanting you to gain weight?" To be honest, it's the closest I came to hitting him. I felt as if he were implying that our mother/daughter relationship was dysfunctional and that somehow I was the cause of her illness.

We were offered "family therapy" to help us work through our "communication issues" and to help me "separate" myself from Molly so that she could function independently. I was so angry and confused by this needless and almost ridiculous emphasis on "family problems". So much so that I'd find myself waking up in the small hours of the night, asking myself if really there was something wrong with the way we had brought Molly up. Had we loved her too much? Was that even possible? In retrospect, I think it was all complete nonsense. We were close and loving before and we are close and loving now. I'm still angry that people made me doubt myself, doubt my husband and doubt us as a couple and as parents.

I am relieved to say that Graham has made a good recovery and is immensely grateful that we lived so close to such a great hospital as Harefield. I think it's ironic that on the one hand we were able to benefit from amazing clinicians who saved my husband's life while with Molly we were very much on our own. I'd love it to be mandatory that in every GP practice there is *at least* one person who understands eating disorders and is up to date with the latest thinking on treating these illnesses. If it's not possible to have one person in every practice, then at least be able to make a swift and informed referral to someone else locally who can help.

Molly has been able to make such an amazing recovery because we were fortunate enough to come across an online resource in F.E.A.S.T. that educated, informed and supported us in making choices that saved her life. At times it felt like a bit of a gamble because we had so little faith in the options being presented by the GP and the local hospital. But, ultimately, we had to trust that, as her parents, we knew best. I certainly wouldn't advocate our approach for everyone, though. If you can work with a team of experienced clinicians who are supportive of Family-Based Treatment, and who see you as part of the solution rather than part of the problem, you are very fortunate and have a huge advantage.

Today, Molly looks and feels beautiful. She has bright eyes, shiny hair and lovely curves. She laughs all the time. She is very much loved and she knows that. Most importantly, she has a future which will be happy and healthy. Her experience has changed her, certainly, but probably for the better. She has huge levels of empathy for other people and I believe she knows just how fortunate she is to have survived the hell of anorexia.

MY TIPS:

Take control - and don't be afraid of what your child is afraid of.

Trust your intuition. The experts don't always know as much as you assume they do.

Look after yourself. Once Molly was at a healthy weight, I had a complete breakdown. At Christmas 2011 I visited the doctor and sobbed uncontrollably for a full half hour. I felt as though my life had irreparably changed and all the certainty that had given me such security and confidence before had vanished. I was fearful all the time that something awful was about to happen. I'm not sure how I could have avoided this. People talk about self-care being so important and it really is, but in my case I think I was just too pig-headed to do anything about it. I've always been a very driven person and I was determined to get my family through a very challenging situation. I didn't stop to think about what would happen to me if we got through it

No-one will love or know your child better than you. Don't let anyone knock your confidence or tell you to step back and "leave this to the experts".

Recovery is possible. Don't ever give up and when setbacks occur (and, believe me, they will occur), face them and move on.

Join the ATDT forum. Don't be afraid of the internet or think it's "weird" to form relationships with a group of individuals you've never met before but end up speaking to online at all hours of the day and night. Places like the ATDT forum can provide life-saving support and comfort during what can be a very bleak time. (See list of resources at the end of the book.)

Look after your marriage or relationship. I was totally focused on my daughter, even when my husband was recovering from his heart attack. I rationalised that I knew his life was saved, but I didn't know if we could save Molly, so in my mind this justified cutting Graham out of a lot of things.

You will get your child back. Your relationship with your child may feel terrible for a long time and you may think you won't ever regain their love and trust. But you will. Anorexia makes demons of them. When it's gone, they come back. Molly had a job interview recently and the interviewer asked her to talk about someone she felt was "inspirational". She said "My mum". Every time I think of that comment I feel so grateful and blessed. We love one another so much and, in a way, I'm glad to have been given the opportunity to show her how far I would go and what I would do to keep her safe. This sounds odd I know, but Molly will never be able to doubt the depth and intensity of a parent's love.

Ultimately, I believe food is the answer. Not the whole answer in that there may be underlying co-morbid conditions that need addressing. Low self-esteem needs to be dealt with and often other things too. But food is so important. It is also vital to learn to externalise the illness - in other words to separate the illness from your child, almost as if they were two "beings". Looking back I can see how important it was, too, to deal with the rages and horrible behaviours in a calm, supportive and consistent way. This is definitely easier said than done. In the early days of Molly's illness when I was caring for her full-time at home, I attended four carers' workshops at a big hospital in South London in an effort to upskill myself. They reinforced the idea that I needed to remain calm, consistent and supportive at all times. Even when I felt like screaming. Even when I was being screamed at. This persona was presented as a calm dolphin-like personality who nudges their child along, guiding from the side, always supportive, well balanced and calm.

Don't give up. I haven't yet met a parent that would entertain the idea that their child could have an eating disorder for life. Giving up on your child is never an option because there are so many grounds for optimism. Be frightened by all means; indeed a sense that you are standing on a burning platform can actually spur you into action and give you a reason to be decisive. Be prepared to make a nuisance of yourself, but don't ever give up. Read stories of other people who have made a full recovery and believe completely that it is possible.

Prepare for setbacks and don't be surprised by them. They do happen and they can be hugely discouraging, but they are steps along the way. Every day remind yourself of how much easier things are becoming and look back to when things were at their worst to remind yourself of how far you have come. Every mouthful, every meal completed, every pound gained is a victory. Nowadays when I look at Molly I want to be able to show her to every desperate mum or dad who has just discovered that their child has an eating disorder and say: "This is what recovery looks like!" It may be fragile, but it's real and we are determined to make sure it lasts.

Marianne's story

"'Can you try and eat an apple?' the GP asked. I sat there open-mouthed. Lindy had almost stopped eating by this point. And, anyway, what difference would an extra 40 or 50 calories make?"

Oh my goodness, do I remember the GP's face when I told her I thought my daughter, Lindy, was developing an eating disorder? The GP just seemed to freeze. Then she went all quiet and starting typing rapidly on the computer. Lindy burst into tears and I did all the talking. It was quite bizarre, it really was. No, it wasn't bizarre; it was terrifying because, by this stage, Lindy had virtually stopped eating. Just a little bit of potato each day, no more than a few hundred calories. And the weight was falling off her.

As a child Lindy had never been fussy about food. She'd been a bit underweight as a toddler, but then she'd put on weight. By her teens she was just normal. In fact we were all so very normal - a normal family with a normal background. We ate normally; indeed we ate very healthily. Lindy had a good appetite. She wasn't fussy like a lot of children; she'd eat everything that was put in front of her.

Then in the lower sixth form, aged 17, she developed a Streptococcal throat infection which made her very poorly and made swallowing difficult. She was put on a fluids-only diet for several days. As a result she lost quite a bit of weight. When she recovered she seemed pleased with her new slimmer appearance.

The following spring, she had appendicitis and lost more weight. Afterwards, her weight continued to drop very slightly. I remember telling her that she didn't need to lose weight; she was fine as she was. But she was gradually restricting and cutting things out of her diet. She decided to go vegetarian, but this didn't trigger any alarm bells because she'd gone veggie on and off before. Meanwhile she'd go out running early in the morning and began exercising with a video exercise game. At first I thought it was just to get fit after the illness, so - again - I wasn't too concerned.

It was the January of her upper sixth form year that she began to look even closer at what she was eating. She cut out bread, for instance. But, again, I didn't really notice anything because it was so very gradual. Her boyfriend would try to take her out for meals but she either wouldn't eat or she'd eat very little. Her friends began to pick up on this, although I only found this out recently. "Why didn't you tell me?" I asked them. "We thought you knew!" they said. Her boyfriend was worried, too. But he didn't say anything either.

Looking back, I really wish people had said something to me because it would have reinforced my own concerns and probably made me act sooner. In fact I feel incredibly guilty about not acting sooner. Why didn't it dawn on me what we were dealing with? The thing is you simply don't expect your healthy, happy, food-loving child to get an eating disorder. I guess I hoped it was just a teenage phase that she would grow out of. But she didn't grow out of it.

I'll never forget the night of the school prom. Lindy didn't want to go; she couldn't face the idea of sitting down to a three-course meal. Already she was down to a very small UK dress size, but when she tried on her dress, it just hung off her. She was freezing cold and I noticed how painfully thin her arms and legs were. We had to call my mum round to take in the dress. My mum was very worried too. In the end, Lindy went to the prom, but she texted me all through the evening for reassurance and support, and she came home early.

We began to notice that she was getting pale. She'd claim to have eaten when she hadn't. Lindy had a part-time evening job in a restaurant and she'd have her evening meal there - just half a jacket potato and some beans because she'd "had a big lunch at school".

Then the beans went and it was just the half potato with some salad. I was desperate to understand why she was doing this; I felt she was slim enough. Too slim… But I was scared to say anything in case it made things worse. It's difficult to explain unless you've been through this, but I really felt that by keeping quiet things would eventually change and Lindy would get back to normal.

Having said this, deep down I had a hunch that it was an eating disorder. One day I approached her with: "I think there might be a problem." She just looked at me and said: "I haven't got anorexia."

But over the next few weeks she began to get stomach aches. She'd claim to feel bloated. One evening I remember her lying on the sofa. My husband and I had planned to challenge her about things. She got upset, saying she was in pain. She was crying: "Mum, I think I've got a problem!"

"Oh, Lindy, I am so pleased you've told me!" I told her we'd been going to say something. I said we must go and see the GP and get her checked over. She didn't want to go. "I've noticed you're a bit pale," I said in a bid to get a pretext for going. "You might be anaemic. You might need some iron pills." Her periods had also stopped; so I told her she really needed to get that checked out, too. Thankfully, Lindy agreed to come along. By this time she'd lost over a stone and you could tell. She looked ill. Her face was ice cold. The skin on her cold hands was red and dry. Worse, she was developing fine hair on her face.

So we went to the GP and, as described above, the GP froze. But she did arrange for Lindy to have an ECG and some blood tests. I explained that Lindy was just eating half a jacket potato a day, and that was all. "Can you try and eat an apple as well?" the GP asked her. I sat there open mouthed. I mean, Lindy had almost stopped eating by this point, certainly eating no more than 300 calories a day. Getting her to eat an apple would have been nigh impossible. And, anyway, what difference would an extra 40 or 50 calories make? I remember thinking "The GP has no idea what we're dealing with!" and I panicked. Actually I did more than panic; I began to lose hope.

I think it's because when you go to the GP you expect them to know what the problem is, to scoop you up and winch you to safety. I wanted to hand it over to the GP knowing that she'd sort it out. But she didn't. Don't get me wrong, she was really sympathetic and obviously wanted to help. It's just that she didn't have a great deal of knowledge about eating disorders.

Anyhow, the GP said she'd be away on holiday for the next two weeks but we could come back when she returned. "No, that's too long!" I said, aware that Lindy was losing weight fast. I asked if there was someone else we could see in the meantime.

This time Lindy went alone, with her boyfriend. The GP checked her blood and did an ECG. Everything was normal on that count. Lindy was also weighed, but at this point her weight wasn't dramatically low so the GP didn't appear overly concerned. It also meant that she didn't qualify for Adult Mental Health Services - at 18 she was too old for CAMHS.

Thankfully, through a colleague at work, I'd come across an eating disorders service which was located about 20 miles away, part-funded by the NHS and part-funded by charity. Lindy could either self-refer or get a GP referral. We did both!

Amazingly we only had to wait two weeks before seeing the service - right on top of Lindy's A-level examinations. Also, by this time I knew more about eating disorders. I'd read Janet Treasure's book *Skills-Based Learning For Caring For A Loved One With An Eating Disorder: The New Maudsley Method* and I'd talked to the UK eating disorders charity, Beat.

The eating disorders service was wonderful. Lindy was given a thorough assessment. I was offered support, too, right away. We saw them three times a week. Each time we were there for three or four hours. We'd spend an hour with the dietician, an hour in psychotherapy followed by complementary therapies like reflexology to help Lindy relax after the counselling session. Yes, it was a 40-mile round trip every time we went and it ate up all my days off work, but it was worth it. And to think I would never have heard of this service if it hadn't been for that colleague who mentioned it in passing; the GP never said anything.

I was aware of another, more local eating disorders support service, but Lindy wasn't considered sufficiently sick to be seen by them; her BMI wasn't low enough. If we'd never discovered the other service, what would we have been supposed to do? Wait until she deteriorated sufficiently to get admitted to the local service? It doesn't bear thinking about - especially as, when Lindy began treatment, she'd completely stopped eating. She wasn't eating a thing, just drinking diet coke and black coffee. As you can imagine, I was petrified as to where this was heading. She'd already lost a considerable amount of weight when she was "eating"; now that she'd stopped altogether... well... But even then her BMI wasn't low enough to be referred to the local service, so thank God I'd managed to get her in at the other one.

I remember the day Lindy was officially diagnosed with an eating disorder. We all sat down as a family. Lindy's boyfriend was there as well. He said: "I am so relieved - thank you for doing this for her." I thought, well I haven't done anything! But it was an immense relief to all of us.

At our first session with the dietician, I explained that Lindy had stopped eating. Together we put together an eating plan. We'd start gradually; initially we wanted Lindy to have a smoothie and an *Actimel* each day. It doesn't sound much, but it was a step in the right direction. Of course this wasn't sufficient and she continued to lose weight. Meanwhile we continued to work with the dietician on a workable re-feeding plan. The dietician would gradually add things and I did a lot of work on it at home.

I remember the time we tried to get Lindy to drink a smoothie one evening. Her dad sat on one side of her while I sat on the other. She cried all the way through. We were still sitting there at 11 o'clock at night, me holding the straw, gently persuading her to take small sips. To her credit she eventually managed it. Then, afterwards, her dad took her out for a walk. The idea was to have a chat; to try and calm her down and distract her. But off she went... striding away down the road, intent on burning off the calories she'd just consumed...

This was a very bleak time when she would only have fluids. On one occasion she lost five pounds in just four days. I was very scared. Eventually we managed to get her to move onto solid foods. However, even then, the obsessive behaviours that seemed to be part and parcel of Lindy's eating disorder meant that the foods weren't "allowed" to touch each other. If they did, she'd have a complete meltdown.

Over time, though, things did begin to improve. It was painfully slow and an experience I wouldn't wish on my worst enemy. To be honest, if she and I hadn't received support from that wonderful eating disorders service, I don't think we would have survived; either of us.

It was also around this time I came across Bev Mattocks' blog: *AnorexiaBoyRecovery*. I'd been Googling around, trying to find more information on eating disorders and I just came across it. The blog was a lifeline. Okay, Bev's child is a boy, but there were so many, many similarities. Here was someone who had been through exactly what we were going through. I made contact with Bev and we are still friends to this day.

Through the blog I found F.E.A.S.T. and its forum, Around The Dinner Table. These days I'm a well know fixture on the ATDT forum and I've made a lot of really good "virtual" friends through it. In November 2012 we all met up at a F.E.A.S.T. conference and it was amazing to spend a day with all these people I felt I already knew but had never met!

I have to say that, throughout this time, Lindy's school was fantastic. Remember her treatment had started right on top of A-level examinations? Well, the school gave her the option of not sitting for the exams, but Lindy insisted on going in. She got A-star grades and was offered a place at a top university. Later, however, she made the decision to defer and, eventually, not to take up the place. Again, the school was hugely supportive, helping us to compile a letter to the university and so on.

I remember when Lindy's teachers told me how shocked they were at her diagnosis and how sorry they were that they hadn't recognised what was happening in those early days. Hopefully our experience will help them to pick up on typical signs with other students in the future. But we are truly thankful to the school for its tremendous support once the staff were aware of her illness.

Today, Lindy is almost recovered. There are still a few outstanding glitches, but I think this is only to be expected. She could do with putting on a little more weight, for example. And she still needs occasional help with working out meal plans. But on the whole she is doing very well. She's independent; in fact she and her boyfriend are buying a house together. But I know that if there are any problems, she'll let me know. After all, she and I have been working together as a team; a really successful team, actually. And I continue to be incredibly proud of her strength and determination to recover from this horrible illness - and I let her know how proud I am of her.

MY TIPS:

Get reading. Buy *Skills-Based Learning For Caring For A Loved One With An Eating Disorder: The New Maudsley Method* by Janet Treasure and *Help Your Teenager Beat an Eating Disorder* by David Lock & Daniel Le Grange - both excellent books. (See list of resources at the end of the book.)

Look out for signs. With Lindy these were: cutting down on portions, cutting out carbohydrates, skipping meals, staying in her room, avoiding social situations (especially where food was involved) and not wanting to go to school (she used to love school and in the sixth form she simply went in for lessons and came home. No socialising, no chatting with friends. It wasn't normal. Well, it wasn't Lindy as I'd always known her).

Trust your gut instinct. If you're the slightest bit worried, take your child to see the GP.

Don't let the GP fob you off. If they don't appear to know, then ask your GP if they can find out more about eating disorders, ASAP. This is urgent and, the thing is, you won't believe how quickly they can go downhill once this thing starts. So get your child seen and get them referred. Even if their BMI isn't "low enough", keep insisting on a referral. It's a common myth that, to have an eating disorder, you need to have a skeletal BMI.

Another thing... Write everything down before you visit the GP, especially any changes in behaviour. I used to think that eating disorders were just about "not eating", but they are about so much more - and unusual behaviours (anger, tantrums, depression, self-hatred, self-isolation, etc) are a key part.

Get support for yourself. Visit the F.E.A.S.T. website and Beat (see end of book for links). Join the ATDT forum and introduce yourself to the other parents. Or just have a good read through the posts; you're bound to find another family that is having - or has had - a similar experience to you.

Vicky's story

"It's as if, all of a sudden, my daughter trusts us. She will now let me hug her. She'll talk, she'll chat and she's eating really well. Emotionally our 'little girl' is back with us again. It really is incredible."

Oddly, although I'd been working in mental health for over 20 years, it took me ages before I cottoned onto the fact that my 15-year old daughter, Anna, was developing anorexia. I knew that eating disorders were mental illnesses and that they were difficult to treat, but that was about it. Like many people, I just assumed they happened to other families; not families like ours and certainly not to a lovely, normal girl like our daughter, Anna.

It was January, and I was vaguely aware that Anna had put on a bit of weight over Christmas. She'd gone on a diet. She didn't lose much, just a few pounds. I didn't think anything of it. Well, you just don't, do you? Then along came Lent and I noticed that Anna was becoming very strict with herself. She gave up everything: chocolate, cakes, biscuits, sweets, puddings… I remember thinking how incredibly strong willed she was being. I probably even admired her. But, again, she didn't lose that much weight so the alarm bells didn't go off.

Then, in April, Anna had an operation under general anaesthetic. There were complications and she was quite poorly afterwards, so she wasn't eating very much. I was taking meals into the hospital for her at that point. But I put the lack of appetite down to the fact that she'd had a general anaesthetic and wasn't feeling too good.

When she came home, she wore baggy sweatshirts and jogging bottoms, even to school. She was in a wheelchair or on crutches, so casual clothes were easier to wear. Again, I still wasn't too worried about the seeming lack of appetite as she wasn't using up much energy in the wheelchair. It wasn't until later when she got back into her school uniform and I saw her in her skirt and tights that I remember thinking: "Oh my goodness, she's lost so much weight!" I actually said to her: "Anna, you've lost too much weight!" I told her that we were going back to normal eating.

But things weren't normal. One day I baked a carrot cake. I gave her a piece and I saw her put it back in the cake tin. I remember thinking: "We've got a real problem here." Crucially, it didn't take ages to get to this point; it all happened really quickly. One night I'd been out with friends. I'd had a bit to drink and decided to say something because it had been praying on my mind all evening. I went into Anna's bedroom and she was still awake. She had her headphones on and I asked her why. She said she couldn't sleep without them. I responded with: "I think you've got an eating disorder." She started to cry and said: "I'm so scared mum, I'm so afraid." To be honest, if she hadn't admitted that there was something up… if she'd said something like: "Oh I'm fine, mum," I would probably have ignored it. You see, she'd only lost about 12 pounds.

I immediately rang some friends whose daughter had had anorexia and said: "What do I do?" We went down to see them that weekend. They gave me some books and the direct number for our local eating disorders service. I called the lead clinician who said he'd see us within the week. I heard nothing, so I hassled. And I continued to hassle until I got an appointment a few days later.

Thankfully we were fortunate in that we could self-refer to a specialist NHS eating disorders team, without going through our GP. Also, I work in mental health, so I was probably able to use my connections to get an appointment quickly. In a way I'm relieved we didn't go down the GP route because, about two months later, I went to the GP to ask for some antidepressants. I was finding it hard to cope. He asked why I wanted the medication and I said: "Because my daughter's got anorexia." So he asked me how thin she was. I said she'd got a BMI of 18.5 and he responded with: "Well, she sounds fine to me." I was stunned.

Initially Anna, who is now 16, saw a psychiatrist - a general psychiatrist, not an eating disorders specialist. To be truthful, I wasn't that impressed. But then we switched to a specialist therapist who was very good. He'd worked in eating disorders for 20 years or so. We saw him for a few months and we've been seeing two further therapists ever since, both of whom are good.

Now that Anna is improving, we only see them once a fortnight. The treatment is going well. We have our blips, but she's now weight restored; in fact she was weight restored at Christmas. Mind you, it took the threat of hospital admission to get her there. We had some extremely difficult times. The pivotal moment took place in the hospital coffee shop. We'd been sitting there with the consultant psychiatrist, discussing getting Anna sectioned. Faced with the prospect of being admitted, something must have "clicked" inside Anna's head, and slowly things began to improve from that moment on.

These days Anna is doing well. She doesn't like talking about her eating disorder, mind you. She doesn't like anyone talking about it and so we avoid the subject. Anna is doing things her own way and I believe she will succeed. She hates going to therapy. In fact she hasn't used it in any way; it's been my husband and I that have used it. The good news is that she's started to talk a little. I still think there are things that she needs to talk about and she realises this. We are here, whenever she feels the need to open up, which she does sometimes in therapy sessions. Surprisingly for someone with anorexia, she's never lied to us. Sometimes she doesn't have lunch and she brings it back from school untouched, but she's very honest about it.

But I'm still annoyed with myself that, although I work in mental health and have done so for 20 years, I didn't pick up on Anna's emerging anorexia. I certainly had no idea that there was an "emotional" angle to the illness and that it could be so extreme: things like parent-hatred, depression and distressing behaviour. I wasn't aware that there were "voices", either. In other words it's as if "something" is talking to your child inside their head, telling them not to eat and telling them they are fat.

During the worst period, Anna's behaviour could be really extreme. For at least two months she spat at me every time she saw me. She wouldn't come into the kitchen if we were in there. She was too terrified, so we had to leave a meal on the table for her. She ate it, but we had a lot of issues with emotional anorexia. Even now, ten months on, she won't sit in the front seat of the car with me and she won't let me touch her. The other month, for example, we were having a really nice chat. She was about to get a coach to Newcastle and I thought: "Ooh, I'll give her a hug goodbye." So I hugged her and she totally recoiled. A few minutes later I got a got a text saying: "Don't you ever touch me again." It was heart-breaking.

The good news is that, throughout all this, Anna has hardly missed a day of school. She's doing really well and has managed to keep her friendship group. Her friends have been great. She hasn't been easy to be with, but her friends have been lovely. In fact she's functioning reasonably well on most fronts with the exception of the particular issue she seems to have with me. It's getting easier, but it's still there. It's very distressing, as you can imagine. But the other half of me says: "Well, she's eating and she's weight restored, so I need to count my blessings." In fact the eating bit came together very quickly which we were relieved about.

Anna is the youngest of three children. My eldest daughter, who is 20, works in Leeds. She found Anna's illness hard to deal with and got quite upset when it was at its worst. But she's been really supportive and calls me every day to ask how it's going. She has also been very supportive to Anna which is really great.

My son, who's 18 and on a gap year, was around during the worst period. He was brilliant; he just "got it". He was very empathetic and knew exactly what to say and when. To be honest, he was better than any of us. He emailed her all the time from wherever he happened to be and when things were at their worst he'd say: "It's all right, mum, she'll get through it." He's planning to study medicine and I am sure he'll make a very sensitive doctor especially as he is thinking of specialising in psychiatry.

As a parent, you really do need the support of other people who "get it". I went along to a local self-help group for parents of young people with eating disorders which I found helpful. Also, a couple of months into Anna's illness, I came across the F.E.A.S.T. website and the Around The Dinner Table forum. ATDT has been a bit of a lifesaver. You see, it's all well and good going along with your child to therapy once a week for 60 minutes, but you're talking about getting them to eat; there's precious little time to talk about the emotional side of things - the parent-hatred, the meltdowns and all that. So it's essential for parents to get support for themselves. Having said this, I've come to the point where I'm thinking that I need to break away from it all; to put all this behind us and move on.

Hopefully, with the help of Anna's therapists, the remaining issues will come together over the coming months. More than anything I long to give my daughter a big hug and for her to hug me back. Yes, I think I look forward to that more than anything.

MY TIPS:

Talk to your child. If you suspect that something is up, then do ask your child if they are struggling with their eating. They may well deny there is a problem at first, but you will still get a reaction if you have touched a nerve. That's how we confirmed there was a problem.

Eating disorders are serious illnesses. Please seek effective treatment fast and don't let anyone fob you off.

Educate yourself about the illness. If you know of anyone who has been through this go and talk to them. We were fortunate to have some friends who had been dealing with this for two years, and they opened our eyes to the seriousness of the condition, gave us advice about how to start re-feeding treatment, and gave us lots of books to read.

Read, read, read. Register with the F.E.A.S.T. eating disorders website; they have an excellent reading list as well as a plethora of other invaluable resources. (See list of resources at the end of the book.)

Take this very seriously. Be prepared to put your life on hold. Time off from work will be needed and it is worth speaking to your employer about this. If possible, have two adults at home in those difficult first few weeks. You are likely to meet with a great deal of resistance and anger.

Talk to others in your child's life and get them on board: teachers, sports coaches, your child's friends and parents of friends. Be aware that your child may not want many people to know; our daughter only told three close friends, but these friends and their parents were invaluable in providing feedback and support to us, and support to our daughter during her illness.

Set incentives. For our daughter the important motivator in her life was sport. We stopped all sport, but allowed it to be slowly reintroduced with each target weight gain. When things became unmanageable at home, hospital admission was clearly spelt out as a consequence if things did not improve. Similarly we used calls to the police, use of a home treatment team and other things to show that there were consequences for unacceptable behaviour.

Be open-minded about the use of medication to help your child. During treatment when we came to a standstill, we felt medication would be helpful, but we had to push for this.

Establish routines for meals. In retrospect we should have been more forceful early on in establishing routines such as sitting at the table to have breakfast. We managed to establish reasonably good routines for other meals, but allowed our daughter too much freedom in getting her own breakfast and eating away from the table. As a consequence we never felt we had full control over the amount of food Anna consumed at breakfast.

Insist on 100% weight restoration. Initially the therapist set a target weight that was too low - only 95% of weight restoration. We later insisted on 100% weight restoration but as the earlier target had already been set - in front of our daughter - it made the job of setting the revised target weight harder. My advice would be to discuss the target weight privately with your therapist and be assertive if you feel it is too low.

Don't be afraid to constantly challenge the eating disorder. It can be hard, and exhausting, but it helped us to make progress. In other words, don't "collude" with it - or attempt to rationalise with it. You will gradually realise when it's your "real child" who is talking and when it's the eating disorder.

Eating disorders love triangulation. All adults involved in your child's treatment need to present a united front. It's true what they say about the illness being very devious and manipulating differences between you and your partner. We worked hard at staying together by regularly giving each other feedback and talking about strategies.

Be kind to yourself and seek support. Often our treatment sessions were more about supporting us than our child, mainly because we had reached the stage where we were exhausted and couldn't cope. So if you need help, ask.

We found that arranged holidays or other events were a major source of stress. As the event approached, we had to decide whether to cancel or go. Either answer was wrong as Anna felt responsible for cancelling our holiday or for us not going to events. Or when we did go it inevitably proved very difficult. So we eventually got to the stage where we didn't arrange anything, and that was better and less stressful. Our advice would be to wait until you are really sure you can go, and only then arrange it.

Be patient. Recovery takes a long time. Don't give up hope.

POSTSCRIPT - by the author

A month or so after talking to Vicky, I received an email. "Hi Bev, Would you like me to add a bit to my story? Anna is now allowing me to cuddle and kiss her - 11 months after all this began! And she's engaging with her therapist and feeding herself independently. In fact I'd say we are NEARLY there!!!"

So I called Vicky right back to find out more.

"Three weeks ago, Anna started on medication," Vicky explained. "I don't know if it's this that's responsible for the improvement. Or the fact that, following a particularly bad session with the psychiatrist, I sided with Anna and told her that if she didn't want to see him again then this was perfectly okay with me. However I told her that I'd be putting all my trust in her to agree to work with me instead. And, you know, it just changed things!"

In the event, Vicky and Anna are still receiving help. "We've switched to a different psychiatrist but we're still seeing the same therapist who is hugely supportive. It's as if, all of a sudden, Anna trusts us. She will now let me hug her. She'll talk, she'll chat and she's eating really well. I think the medication has helped; I think it's just lifted her mood that little bit, but she may have got there anyway - it's difficult to tell."

Vicky explained that Anna has been suffering from Post-Traumatic Stress Disorder - flashbacks to the stressful re-feeding period. "But she's opening up about this in therapy, so we can move forward," Vicky continued. "She's being referred to a specialist in PTSD. I feel grateful that we have a resource locally that can deal with this. Anna is doing just fine; she's really great. Emotionally our 'little girl' is back with us again. It really is incredible!"

Emma's story

"These days, she'll come in with a takeout, just like anyone else. She'll grab a burger here and a pizza there, or sit down in front of the telly with a tub of ice cream. She is just a really happy young lady."

Amber had always been a quiet child, preferring a small circle of friends. She was happy, but she'd always had what I can only describe as an air of sadness about her. We put it down to her being thoughtful and quiet. Amber was Amber, happily plodding along through life, head in the clouds and a bit of a dreamer.

She'd never had any issues with food and had always eaten healthily. She was never fussy and never picky. My husband works from home so he would always cook the dinner which Amber and her younger sister, Jade, would eat without any problem. She was a keen club swimmer, training several times a week. She enjoyed swimming but she was never fast enough to swim competitively. As a child, she wasn't tiny; she was always at the top of her growth chart and quite tall. She was just a normal child - neither skinny nor fat, just average.

Looking back in hindsight, Amber wasn't the typical stereotype for classic anorexia, either, in that she wasn't a high achiever. She was, and still is, a very bright girl with a string of exam passes but she has always been content to sit back and do "just enough" to get by.

When she was eight Amber was tested for early onset puberty. Everything came back okay. But it could be that, from this point on, she began to think she might be different from the other girls. By the age of 10 or 11 she was one of the tallest girls in the year and she started saying that she didn't like her body very much. There was also a bit of bullying that went on in year 6 with some of the other girls - the "cool kids" she called them - and I think there was a bit of pushing and shoving, that kind of thing. She never really spoke too much about it, and Amber and her friends eventually learned to ignore the bullies.

Then when she went to senior school in year 7, she started her periods and, obviously, everything started to grow. Amber didn't like her new boobs. We're quite a voluptuous family and she didn't like it. Then she started saying: "My head's too small for my body." "Disproportionate" was the word that kept cropping up.

By the time she went into year 9 there still wasn't anything to set off the alarm bells. But every so often I'd catch her looking at herself in the mirror. She'd complain that her head was too small, that she was out of proportion or that she didn't like her body. So I'd say, "You're just going through puberty. Once you've finished growing everything will balance out". She also stopped swimming at this time as the training sessions were increasing in frequency and began to interfere with her schoolwork. As a result, she lost some muscle tone. I often wonder if this could have been a trigger for the eating disorder.

Year 10 was the year they chose their GCSE subjects. It was also the year that things started to go downhill. Amber had two close friends, both boys, and both emigrated within a couple of months of each other. Amber really missed them. Also, her choice of GCSE options meant that she wasn't in classes with any of her other friends. She became depressed, and that's when it all began.

Just days after starting Year 10 in September 2008, Amber began to push her food around the plate at evening meals. I was working late every night, often not getting back until after everyone had eaten, so initially I wasn't aware of this.

We also had no idea that she was getting up at the crack of dawn, going downstairs before any of us were up, putting a few crumbs of cereal and a splash of milk into a bowl and saying that she'd had her breakfast. Then she'd take her packed lunch to school and throw it away. But, at the time, we didn't know this was going on; it was only much later, when her worried best friend's mother told me what she was doing, that it all came to light.

Back home in the evening, my husband would put dinner in front of her. She'd eat half of it and say, "I'm too upset to eat". She was really missing her two male friends. Well, we just told her not to worry, she'd get through it and it would all turn out fine.

It got to the October half term. By then I'd left my stressful job and gone freelance, so I was home for dinner at a more regular time each evening. We were due to go to Barcelona for a week with my closest friend and her children and were packing to go. Amber said, "I need new jeans, mum". So I asked her why; we'd only bought new ones a few weeks ago. She said they didn't fit her any longer. My initial reaction was, okay, she's obviously grown; she needs the next size up. So I told her we'd go shopping for a bigger size.

"But I don't need a bigger size," she said, "I need a smaller size". Well, I looked at her and she was standing in her bedroom wearing opaque black tights and black shorts, like girls do. It was if a veil was suddenly lifted from my eyes. I thought: "Oh my God, Amber, what have you done?" It looked as if she had two strings of liquorice hanging out of her shorts.

"Right, on the scales," I said immediately. So I got out the scales and discovered that she'd lost a stone. I was shocked. I said: "What have you done? I know you've been upset but you mustn't lose weight because of it."

It never even crossed my mind that she was sick. So we went away on holiday and the changes became more and more apparent because we were in close quarters all the time. She'd sit at breakfast saying, "I can't eat this, I'm not hungry, I feel sick". Lunch would be in a restaurant and she'd sit for ages trying to find something to eat. In the end it would be an omelette or something like a simple green salad. As for evening meals… All of a sudden, because we were with her 24/7, it dawned on us that there was a problem.

I'll never forget the day we went to a theme park. Although it was October it was still reasonably warm. We were queuing for a ride when Amber looked at me and said she didn't feel well. She passed out. She simply collapsed in the queue and my husband had to pick her up and carry her out. Once she came to she said, "Dad, I'm fine," and told us all to go back on the ride. But the moment she stood up, she passed out again. She was taken to a medical centre, next to the theme park, and hooked up to a drip. The nurses looked at her and remarked: "She's extremely thin..."

I said that I knew this and told them how much weight she'd lost recently. So they looked at her and said, "You've lost too much weight. You have to put it back on". My husband came in at that point and I think this was his dawning moment, the realisation that this was his "little girl", lying there, so pale and thin, hooked up to that drip. Our younger daughter Jade also came in. As soon as she saw her big sister she burst into tears. By now we were in no doubt that we had a serious problem on our hands.

I remember crying with my close friend: "What on earth am I going to do? Do you think Amber's getting anorexia?" Meanwhile Amber promised us that she'd try to eat. By this stage she had missed two periods but, at the time, I put it down to stress.

Back home we didn't take her to the doctor immediately because we were worried it might make things worse. So, instead, we tried to make her eat. I did give the GP a call, however, and filled her in on what had happened. I told her that Amber had lost a lot of weight, that she'd been very depressed and I didn't know what to do. I think I was still trying to avoid saying, "I think my daughter's got anorexia or an eating problem".

Our GP was lovely. Her initial reaction was to agree with me that Amber was probably suffering from stress and depression. She said that she'd written it all down in her notes and asked us to monitor Amber for a month. If things got worse, then we must bring her straight in. So we spent November trying to avoid the obvious and trying to get her to eat. At this point I was getting up in the morning and making sure I was downstairs before Amber. I'd also contacted the school and told them there might be a problem. By now, the Head of Year had noticed Amber's weight loss and change in personality and wanted to do everything she could to help. They allowed Amber to come home for lunch. We only live half a mile away, so my husband would stop work, pick her up, make sure she had her lunch and then take her back to school for the afternoon session. But despite desperately trying to stop the weight loss, Amber's weight was still going down. We were puzzled. We had no idea that she was getting up in the middle of the night to do sit-ups in her room, so that was obviously affecting the weight. But at mealtimes she would sit there and I would see her eating, so I thought things must be improving. To be honest we were still in a kind of denial, yet deep down I think we knew what was happening.

We saw the GP again in December. Amber had lost another half stone and the GP put her on antidepressants which didn't really make any difference. She was becoming more and more withdrawn, more and more psychologically ill and pulling away from us.

The GP asked us to come back in a week. It was literally just before Christmas. I'd been doing some research on the internet and I'd found Laura Collins' book: *Eating With Your Anorexic*. I cried buckets over it! Even today I still get teary when I think back to this time because it's still so emotionally raw. As a mother, it never heals.

I know now that parents aren't to blame for their child's eating disorder. But back then I racked my brains trying to figure out where we'd gone wrong. I couldn't understand it. Our family was loving, kind and caring. We'd never had any problems and we weren't dysfunctional in any way. Yet even though I know that we weren't at fault, I can't help feeling guilty that I didn't insist on a referral sooner, especially after reading Laura's book and realising what we were up against.

I can honestly say that our doctor was the best GP you could have wished for. She saw us through all of this. All three of us went back to the GP just before Christmas. Amber was still losing weight and by this time she was also uncommunicative. I said: "This isn't just depression; I know she's got anorexia." I told the GP that I knew wholeheartedly what we are dealing with and that Amber needed a referral. We live quite close to a major hospital in south London which has a specialist eating disorders service, so I asked if Amber could be referred there. The GP said she thought this was possible, but Amber would need to go through CAMHS first. So she referred us to CAMHS and asked us to come back after Christmas.

Christmas Eve was the last meal that I can remember she ate properly. It was with all our family. My close friend and her family were there too. Amber just sat there shaking her legs because, by this point, she had the "jiggling legs" where you can't sit still. She would sit on the edge of her seat with her legs going up and down, and I'd put my hand under the table to try and stop them from jiggling. She spent the rest of the day crying on the sofa. Her sobs were endless and gut wrenching; they didn't even sound like normal cries. All she would eat was instant porridge and raspberries. She spent the next three or four days like this. She even thought we were putting calories in the water

Thanks to Laura's book I'd discovered F.E.A.S.T. and its forum Around The Dinner Table. I joined on Christmas Eve. The forum helped us enormously because we knew we weren't alone. I'd put up a post, not knowing what I was going to get back and suddenly there would be a dozen or so other parents who had been through this, all offering support. It was the first time I'd actually put up my hand and said, "Please help me!" and from that point on I knew we weren't alone. We started to follow their advice which was basically to get Amber to eat.

Psychologically, however, Amber was in meltdown. Shortly before Christmas she'd self-harmed using a knife. It was the first time ever that she'd seen her dad cry. Terrified, we hid everything we felt might prove a danger to her. We even took the locks off the bathroom doors. And, because she would scratch herself in the shower, I insisted on sitting with her while she showered. It was as if she'd had a complete breakdown.

By this time Amber was crying continuously from the minute she woke up until the minute she went to bed. This continued for two solid weeks. She slept with me every night until I was so exhausted that I wasn't eating properly either! So my husband and I began alternate night shifts. He said he didn't care if people said anything about sleeping in the same bed as his daughter; sleeping in our arms as she had when she was a baby was the only time she was at peace.

When the time came for our families to return home after Christmas, I remember crying: "Don't leave us! I can't do this by myself!" I needed my mum, I needed my mother-in-law and I needed my sister. So we set up a rota and my sister moved in with us, mainly to look after Jade, because our energies were taken up with feeding Amber.

The moment Christmas was over we took her back to the GP and insisted something was done urgently. The GP said she'd try to speed up the CAMHS appointment. CAMHS called me and an appointment was set for early January.

CAMHS were brilliant. They called me every day. Between us, we all realised how sick Amber was to such an extent that, in the event, she bypassed CAMHS altogether and went straight to the adolescent eating disorders centre at the hospital in south London.

We took her there in early January. She was given an ECG but they couldn't find a heartbeat; her rhythms were so low. They couldn't get blood, either, and her weight was registering as shockingly low. By this time her clothes were just hanging off her, her hair was falling out in clumps and she looked like a skeleton.

It took 40 long minutes to get a vial of blood. I think this is when my husband and I reached our lowest point. Suddenly it hit us - the sheer horror of realising how much weight she'd lost. Yet I just couldn't get her to eat, and there was nothing I could do. I felt so incredibly helpless.

I remember asking the treatment team what we were supposed to do, and they simply said: "She just has to eat." We were to sit with her and try to calmly ensure that this is what she did, even if it took all day. They told us that Amber was severely anorexic but, because she had fallen sick so quickly and got help, they were confident of a full recovery, stressing that the quicker she regained weight and got above their weight criteria, the better the outcome could be. They put her on anxiety medication to calm her, as well as antidepressants and stressed how vital fats were for her malnourished brain. I remember her meal plan was full of full-fat milk, butter and cream!

The illness had her in a stranglehold. She couldn't even feed herself. If I gave her anything to hold, even a spoon, she'd scream and drop it as if it was white hot. So we started to spoon-feed her, just like we used to do when she was a baby. It was heart-breaking.

Oh, Amber would scream and weep; it was like having the exorcist child in the house. Her eyes would change and go dark and hard. We'd watch a curtain come down in her brain. But ultimately, with our help, she did start to eat. I think she knew she was so very ill. And you know why I believe she wouldn't feed herself? Because if we fed her then she could *blame us* for making her "fat"; she wasn't *making herself* "fat", if this makes sense.

She'd resist. She'd refuse to eat. But we persisted. We'd sit with her, chop up the food and persuade her to eat it. I downloaded a mountain of calorie-laden recipes from the F.E.A.S.T. website and put all kinds of things into the other meals: cream, butter and oil, basically making everything as calorific as I could. An American friend sent over tubs and tubs of high calorie instant breakfast drinks and I'd feed Amber ice cream and milkshakes.

Between the January and February, we managed to get a stone back onto her. So she did very well. As she became better nourished, we began to see glimpses of the "old" Amber; not the one who'd been consumed by anorexia. But she still couldn't feed herself. Also, I was horrified to see that, with her new-found strength, she became more vocal and resistant.

One awful day in mid-February I'd gone to school to pick up my youngest daughter, Jade. My sister was here at home. It was snack time, and my husband had given Amber a milkshake or something, but she refused to drink it. Suddenly Amber lashed out and whacked my husband around the face, getting violent and screaming profanities. I walked in with Jade to find my sister, who'd been helping out, sitting on the kitchen floor crying. My husband was in his study with the door shut and Amber was up in her room, rocking on her bed. It was hell.

At the time we were visiting the hospital three times a week. At first Amber would just sit there glaring at her therapist through her fringe and muttering. But, as she began to regain some weight and her brain became better nourished, she began to engage with him more. He explained that, once she was more weight restored, he could begin the real work of therapy.

Amber's therapist would ring us on the days we didn't attend to make sure everything was okay. When we told him about the violence, he said, "Bring her in, bring her food and we'll sit behind two-way glass and watch what she does". So this is what we did. There, in the hospital, my sister and I tried desperately to get Amber to eat a sandwich and feed herself a yoghurt, which she found virtually impossible. She sat there holding the spoon in her shaking hands, unable to put it in her mouth, before screaming and throwing it to the floor, while they watched. Our words of encouragement that she could do this were met with swearing and screaming: "I know I can do it, I just *don't* want to!" This was when they said she needed to be admitted to a specialist unit.

They made a phone call and got her into a specialist adolescent eating disorder unit on the other side of London. It was miles away from where we live, but they insisted it was the best place for her. She went pretty much the next day.

I think she thought we'd never do it, that we'd never leave her in that unit. And it still affects her to this day. If she carries any scars from this period I think it's that we took her and left her there.

I'll never forget the day we took her along. My husband put her suitcase in the car. She was screaming and crying because she didn't want to go. She was holding onto the door. My husband had to literally pick her up and put her into the car. That was just, oh, so very hard. But we did it. I have never felt so heartbroken or alone as I did at that time.

Thankfully the unit wasn't like a hospital at all. It was an old house. It was cheerfully decorated and felt quite homely. But I couldn't help noticing that it had bars on the windows and so on.

But, really, they were lovely. The nursing staff and the doctors were great and Amber made some good friends, several of whom she is still in touch with today. And they're all mostly doing okay.

When she was admitted, she was actually in a better state of health than a lot of the children that were there and for that reason she'd keep saying to us: "I don't belong here! I'm not like the other girls. I'm bigger than the other girls so I can't be that ill. I don't need to be here!" And she'd repeat this every night when we visited. It broke my heart. And I was just so very, very tired. After all we were doing a 140-mile round trip every night through some of London's worst motorway traffic. It became a routine. We'd set off at around 4pm and usually arrive for around 6pm so we could eat dinner with her. Then we'd have to leave at 9pm and could arrive home at anything up to 11 o'clock at night. It was a tough time.

I had to laugh, because people would tell us that having your child in hospital is a good opportunity to take time out for yourself, to rest and recharge your batteries. But, for us, we were working all day, sorting out our other daughter and spending up to four hours travelling through busy traffic - and then spending around three hours every evening with Amber. On the rare days when we didn't visit we would be on the phone with her all evening because she was lonely. It was very, very hard. But we did it, because that's what parents do. And we were desperate for Amber to get well.

Another thing that cut me to the core was the fact that this was one of the first times that Amber had ever been away from home on her own for any length of time, apart from school trips and sleepovers. I didn't want this for my daughter. It was devastating for us, especially for me, to take her and leave her there. It was the hardest thing I've ever done.

Every single night I'd arrive home with a broken heart. Because it's not as if we'd left her in a unit around the corner; we'd taken her 70 miles away and left her in the care of others. The guilt was immense. I felt as if I couldn't care for her; as if I'd failed to make her well on my own and that I had to leave her with other people to do this. But the other part of me understood that she was in the best place because, from that point on, she started to eat by herself.

In fact she'd actually started to feed herself the day before we took her there. I think she felt that she had to prove to us that if she could do it, then she wouldn't have to go to the unit. Suddenly she'd say: "I can do it, mum! Look, I'm eating for myself! So I don't need to go there!" And we'd reply with, "Well, you do need to go there, but we'll come and see you every day," which is what we did.

In the unit, Amber was eating. She was doing everything she could to get better. She just wanted to be at home. She graduated from 24/7 care, where she was watched around the clock, even while asleep, to visits where we could take her out for a drive or even eat a meal or a snack with just us and no carers in attendance. After a couple of weeks, she was also allowed to come home for the weekend.

Around Easter, after Amber had been there for five weeks, we went in for an assessment and they told us they felt she was getting more depressed being away from us than she would be back at home. And, because she'd put on another stone or so, they said they'd discharge her and refer her back to the hospital in south London where she continued with twice-weekly sessions which, as time went on, reduced to once a week.

Amber also went back to school. She hadn't been there since Christmas. The school was wonderful. They said they could arrange for tutors to teach her at home - or the tutors could come into school and work with her in the library. Amber preferred being in school, so this is what happened. At this time she was only doing mornings and she wasn't in classes. Everyone - from the form tutors through to the heads of year - was totally and utterly fantastic. They were completely supportive of her right up to when she left at the end of the upper sixth form. We managed to get a "statement" from the local educational authority on medical grounds which allowed the school to pay for a Special Education Assistant to help her with catching up on lessons and taking notes. This allowed her to take her exams on a computer in the special education unit because she found it much easier to type than to hold a pen. She also had extra time in exams because her concentration levels were not as they should be for a girl of her age.

In year 11, her GCSE year, Amber began to do full days. One of us would go in at break and sit with her while she had her snack and her friends would try to make sure she ate all her lunch. Meanwhile, despite the odd month where her weight would drop slightly, she continued to gain. Also, it was around this time that, after fifteen months, her periods returned. But the minute Amber's weight dropped below a certain point they'd switch off again. She came to judge this as her "cut off point" where she couldn't go any lower. And she'd agree with me: "Okay I need to have an extra drink or an extra snack to bring the weight back up again." She was truly awesome, because I was well aware of how hard this was for her. I was so very, very proud of my daughter.

It was a very long time before she stopped saying things like, "Well, I can only eat *this* for my snack" or "I can only have *that* from the meal plan". It was also a while before she stopped insisting on low fat products, for instance low fat yoghurts as opposed to creamy Greek yoghurts, and substituting lower calorie items for the items on the meal plan which the hospital had given her.

I would never have dreamed that one day we would look back on some of the things that went on then and laugh about it - for example her indignation at being given high calorie "ready meals" instead of home cooking. Also the fact that, in her mind, a bowl of soup and a marmite sandwich constituted *two* lunches, not one. However if I took the marmite out, she would eat it!

Amber's therapist at the hospital was excellent. One particular thing I remember him saying was: "You have to pick the battles, as long as she's eating and she's eating everything you're asking her to eat." By this he meant that if she was picking a 90 calorie cereal bar as opposed to 150 calorie one, then that was fine as long as she was eating everything else. Importantly, this wasn't the same thing as allowing her to actively cut back. The thinking was that the odd lower calorie item wasn't a problem as long as she was eating all the other things without a fight.

One thing that made me kick myself, however, was the fact that at Christmas we'd bought the girls a video exercise game which came with its own exercise board. The game measured height and weight and came up with a BMI level which informed my youngest daughter that she was overweight! Immediately I thought: "Oh my God, what have I done!" Especially when Amber began to say things like: "I can't go out. I can't do this or that; I've got to do my exercise." She was addicted to it from the start.

So again the therapist said: "Pick your battles. If she's doing the video exercise game and that's enough for her then at least she's not getting up at 4am and doing a thousand sit-ups that you don't know about. As long as it's not excessive. And, anyway, the endorphins will be good for her." He said that it would go, it would disappear. And it did. Gradually over time we realised that she hadn't done the video exercise that day. And then it would be a week. But before this I felt like the worst mother in the world just sitting there on the sofa watching her jumping up and down on that confounded white board.

The obsessive compulsive tendencies she had developed began to disappear, too. For example she would stand for hours rather than sit down on a sofa where the cushions weren't stacked at exactly the right angle.

Now, four years after this, Amber is fine. She is absolutely fine. Yes, she'll still beat herself up over things and there's still a certain amount of stuff going on in her head. She's still on medication, but these days we no longer weigh her. Her weight is normal, everything is normal. She's perhaps a little shorter than she would have been if she hadn't been ill during puberty but the doctors aren't concerned about osteoporosis or any lasting damage to her bones, which is a huge relief.

I think that now she probably realises that she is no different from anyone else, from any normal girl. Everybody has days where they don't like the look of themselves or they feel down. She has these days, too.

Amber isn't as close as she once was with the childhood best friends who'd overseen her school lunches back in year 11. To be honest, I think they'd found it really hard acting as her "food police" and watching her going through the illness. I think they found it difficult to cope. They and Amber's other friends found it hard to "get" what was going on especially during the period where Amber had gained weight but was still behaving strangely. Doubtless they were thinking: "Well if she *looks* fine then why isn't she *behaving* fine?" Amber felt unable to really talk about what had happened and felt somewhat guilty about what she had put herself and her friends through. I don't think she really felt supported enough, but they were all so very young and ill-equipped to deal with such a devastating illness.

Amber was encouraged through her therapy to push herself to expand her social circle and make new friends. She flitted around for a while between different groups. But, through this, she met a couple of girls who went to a different school. They became her best friends and still are to this day. So much so that these girls actually transferred to Amber's school after the GSCE exams, so they all went through sixth form together. Seeing my beautiful, healthy, brave daughter having a laugh with her friends, just like any other young woman, means more to me than you can possibly imagine. Looking back, we've been so very fortunate. As our therapist said, Amber's eating disorder was caught early. We were also fortunate enough to have treatment at that hospital in south London.

I often look back to that terrible Christmas. I'd just given Amber some spaghetti on toast and she was in meltdown because it wasn't a particular brand of low fat spaghetti and I had added extra butter to it. It was at that moment that the guy from CAMHS called us on the phone. He could hear everything and there I was, crying down the phone to him, "She just won't eat!" It was then that he made the immediate decision to liaise with our GP and the hospital and get her admitted direct rather than bother with the CAMHS route.

If he hadn't done that, well, I don't know if Amber would still be here.

She was so very, very poorly. I remember her smelling strange. Her skin had a yellow tinge. She was covered in dark brown hair all over her body and face. Her hair was falling out in clumps. It was as if everything was shutting down. I remember the terrifying feeling of helplessness. How could she have become that sick so quickly? That's the eye-opening thing about eating disorders; they start very gradually, almost creeping up on you unawares and then - ping! - they're off at a horrendous pace. The momentum was hideous. I am so grateful to that guy at CAMHS for calling at that moment.

Do I have any niggles about Amber's therapy? The hospital were great. They supported her for 18 months through school and through her GCSE examinations. But, because she wasn't technically in any danger at that point and her weight was well above the "danger zone", they signed her off. And that was that. It was all a bit sudden. I felt as if we'd been cast adrift and it was quite unsettling. Also, Amber missed her therapist as he had been so helpful to her.

Looking back, I am certain that she should have been signed back to CAMHS and the GP so she could have been monitored, but she wasn't. As a result we went through 18 months or so in limbo. I think we slipped through the net.

I took Amber back to our GP - a new one, because the original GP had retired - and she said she'd keep an eye on her. She was really good, but Amber wasn't getting any formal therapy. I signed her up with a local free counselling service for teens but she said that, although the counsellor was very nice, she wasn't a therapist and all she did was listen, without treating.

Amber began to get very stressed in the sixth form with the pressure of studies. One day she came to me and told me she was worried that things were getting bad again. She was getting stressed out about her A-levels. My heart sank. So we went straight back to the GP who referred her back to CAMHS who immediately got in touch for an assessment. She was given a six month course of CBT which was really helpful. They signed her off in the August after her 18th birthday. So we had a few months where things were a bit tricky. But thankfully it didn't affect Amber's eating in any way.

These days she's so much happier. She'll come in with a takeout Chinese meal, just like anyone else. Or she'll grab a burger here and a pizza there, or sit down in front of the telly with a tub of ice cream. She is just a really happy young lady.

She laughs easily. She loves a joke with her dad and her sister. She's got a lovely disposition; she's very friendly and her confidence has come back. Also, she's becoming more and more independent, doing things that I never thought I'd see her do - like taking the train into central London where she has a part-time job which she loves. She's taking a year out before continuing her studies which I must admit is a relief because I don't think she would have been able to cope with university and living away from home.

Okay, she'll squabble with her sister, Jade, like siblings do, usually over clothes, hair products and shoes! But this is so very, very normal. The two of them have an excellent bond although my youngest seems older in so many ways. I think it's because all the trauma we've been through forced her to grow up so quickly. As for Amber, well, I think her brain is busy catching up with development as it continues to heal. It's almost like having twins instead of a five-year age gap.

But apart from that, my daughter really is just like any other girl in her late teens. It's almost as if she's picked up where she left off four years ago. It all feels so incredibly normal. But it's taken a heck of a long time to get to this normal. I am so very proud of her and the way she refused to give in to the eating disorder.

Eating disorders don't just affect the sufferer, they affect the family too. Our youngest daughter, Jade, found it particularly hard; in fact she ended up having to have some therapy herself. When Amber first became ill, Jade was only nine years old. She thought her sister was going to die. She felt abandoned because we were constantly focusing on Amber.

In fact I carry a lot of guilt that I might have neglected Jade when she was upset and confused over her sister's illness. I don't believe I ever did neglect her but "mummy guilt" is still with me regardless. I am so proud of Jade for her understanding and her fierce protectiveness over her sister.

I often think how fortunate I was in that all my family were in a position to help. They live an hour or so away from us and were with us constantly during the dark times. My sister, who is ill with ME, set up home with us for almost six months to be there for us all but especially for Jade. Not having children of her own, she has an incredibly strong bond with both her nieces. I can't thank my family enough for their devotion to my children, especially Jade who found it so hard to come to terms with her big sister's illness.

Life goes on in our family and has its normal ups and downs. Sometimes my intuition senses that things are not right, but usually it's down to other teenage problems.

I am trying very hard to step back and let go, but it's difficult. As a parent you are hardwired to nurture and protect, and my beautiful daughter so very nearly died. So there's guilt there, too, even though I know that parents are not to blame for their child's eating disorder.

I would like to be able to say that we are completely out the other side of this dreadful illness, but I can't say we are truly there yet. I don't think we will ever be able to leave it totally behind. I will always be worried. My radar is on constant alert.

I was rocked recently with a revelation from Amber about

vomiting. She was ill a few weekends ago, following a boozy night out and decided that if she made herself sick, she might feel better. She told me in the morning that she had used her bulimic tricks to make herself vomit. When I responded that she'd told me she'd never done that during her illness, she looked at me and simply said… "I lied, I used to do it all the time".

I was shocked because for the last four years I had been taken in and totally believed that lie. I now find myself watching and wondering again, and racking my brains to see if I can remember when she could have possibly done this over the last four years without me noticing. I find myself making excuses to check on her and hover near the bathroom once more. I believe in my heart that she did this when she was early in recovery, probably when she went back to school and was eating on her own. I am certain that she did this out of the house as I would have known and certainly would have found and smelt the evidence, but there was nothing.

I hope and pray that Amber won't ever suffer a relapse. She remains on antidepressants and when she says she is fine, I have to believe her.

Anorexia changed her and changed me. It totally devastated us at the time. We were lucky we had never had to face such trauma in our family before, but it has taught me that we are a strong family, stronger than I ever thought possible. We faced one of the most awful illnesses imaginable and hopefully kicked it out of her life and our lives forever. A telling time will be when Amber eventually leaves home, but thankfully that is still a few years away as the college she hopes to attend is in London. Her healing can carry on at home for now.

I think it is so important for other families facing what we went through to know that it's possible to be a happy family again. You can beat this, just as we did. It will be a long, hard, uphill struggle at times, but you can get there like we did. It just takes endless food, love and patience. And we parents have limitless supplies of that!

Suzie's story

"I explained that we would never let her die, that we loved her and that she was too wonderful to lose. So whether we did it at home, in hospital or through a tube, we would ensure she got the nutrition she needed to get well."

Our story has a happy ending, but only because it was written by the three of us: me, my husband and my beautiful, strong daughter Megan. If we'd left it to the professionals we met along the line I believe the ending could have been altogether different - and it's something that we are still bitter about today.

Before Megan developed anorexia, we were a normal happy family, just like any other family, I guess. Megan was a normal happy kid - the eldest of three children. Life went on as normal until, one day in 2009 when Megan was 13, I noticed a couple of shallow cuts on her arm. When I challenged her about this she claimed to have tripped on the stairs. To be honest, this didn't ring true. So her dad and I began to keep a close watch.

Thankfully nothing else out of the ordinary happened until the summer of 2010, just before Megan's 14th birthday, when we returned from a holiday in France.

As a family we'd always eaten our evening meals together at the table. But, following that holiday, Megan began to leap up from the table and disappear upstairs once the meal was finished. She also made the odd comment about "giving up chocolate" which I thought was odd coming from a child who adored chocolate.

Then the hair pulling began. I'd catch her anxiously tugging at her hair and pulling it out in chunks. Increasingly, she seemed to be finding it difficult to sit still and would constantly jiggle her legs. I thought to myself: "This isn't normal."

We have a set of scales in the bathroom which we rarely use. They began to go missing but no-one in the family would own up to it. So when they were quietly returned we hid them away. But, to be truthful, we didn't think "eating disorder" until the September when Megan went back to school. We felt sure something was up; we weren't quite sure what, but my husband and I were keeping a close watch on things.

I had a chat with Megan's best friend who promised to keep a discreet eye open, too. A week later the friend's mum called to say she'd noticed Megan hiding food in her pockets. Also, they'd gone out for a meal and Megan had been desperate to find a toilet immediately afterwards. "Hmn," we thought, "they're noticing the same things as us". By the end of September we were pretty sure that Megan had an eating disorder.

So we sat her down and told her about our worries. We also told her that she was to sit with us for an hour after every meal, no more running off to the bathroom, and that we'd be giving her three meals and two snacks a day which she must eat. We said: "We love you and we'll get you through this. But first we're taking you to see the doctor so we can all get some professional support."

Looking back I don't know why it took us over a month to take action. It's so easy to wonder if you're imagining things or if it's just regular teenage behaviour. And, of course, you simply don't expect your normal happy child to develop an eating disorder. Anyway, we told the GP about our concerns and asked to be referred to CAMHS. I already knew about CAMHS; as a schoolteacher I often find myself having to refer to them. Fortunately the GP took my concerns seriously and prepared a referral.

He asked a silent Megan to stand on the scales, explaining that she would get through this and would get better. The GP said that some of his fellow students at medical school had suffered from eating disorders. They'd all recovered, so she wasn't to worry. He also told Megan that she must listen to us and that, as her parents, we loved her and knew what was best for her. I remember Megan clinging onto me silently, clearly scared by what was being said.

The CAMHS appointment took five or six weeks to come through. To be honest I was expecting a much longer wait, so this came as a relief. Finally we would be getting professional help.

Meanwhile we were busy trying to re-feed Megan on our own with our three meals and two snacks regime. Thankfully she complied. Or at least she did when she was at home. She was throwing her school lunches away, but I simply made up for this with more calories when she came home. By the time the CAMHS appointment arrived we'd managed to get half a stone onto her.

As a schoolteacher I already knew a bit about eating disorders. Also, as a teenager, I'd had a friend with anorexia who had been treated at a major south London hospital which is well known for its specialist eating disorder services. So I did an internet search for this hospital and read up on everything I could find. I also bought a stack of good books which helped me to learn more about what we were dealing with.

We all went along to CAMHS - me, Megan and my husband. Initially we talked with a nurse therapist who then saw us individually.

And, to be honest, it all went horribly downhill from there.

For a start, I couldn't help noticing that the nurse seemed awfully thin. I don't just mean slim, I mean really skinny. Looking back with the eyes I have now I often wonder if she had an eating issue.

She also seemed quite disturbed that we appeared to know quite a lot about eating disorders. By this time we'd read Janet Treasure's *Skills-based Learning for Caring for a Loved One with an Eating Disorder: The New Maudsley Method* and a host of others. The nurse began to talk about Janet Treasure's animal metaphors (which illustrate the common behaviours and emotional responses of parents of young people with eating disorders). She seemed perturbed to find we were already familiar with these terms.

At one point I said that I believed Megan was purging. And, again, the nurse seemed troubled that we knew what "purging" meant. It was all a bit strange.

Then my husband and I were sent to the waiting area while the nurse chatted to Megan alone. She called us back saying that Megan was a little upset. She'd weighed her (without our permission) and told her what her weight was. If we'd known she was going to weigh her and tell her the weight we would have stopped her.

To make matters worse, the nurse had shown Megan a graph, pointing out that her present weight put her in the 50th centile. She'd informed Megan that this was "completely normal". But Megan is an 85th centile girl; she always had been. So, for us, a 50th centile was quite worrying and scary - and, anyway, she was only up there because we'd yanked her up there through the eating regime.

Of course Megan immediately took this as official confirmation that she was "fat". By the end of the session she was so distressed that she locked herself in the CAMHS toilets. It took me a while to coax her out while the nurse stood to one side, observing.

When we got home, Megan refused to eat. I tried to get her to have a low fat yoghurt. She forced herself to eat a few spoonfuls before rushing to the toilet to throw it back up. I remember her screaming: "I can't do it! I'm not strong enough!"

Over the next fortnight Megan stopped eating and drinking altogether. We were supposed to be seeing CAMHS for a second appointment but we were so worried that, instead, we rushed her down to A&E.

At the hospital Megan was given a brief physical check, but - oddly - she wasn't given anything to eat or drink. We were sent home without any instructions on what we should do. So we struggled on at home for a few more days, without any success.

Five days later we were back in A&E. Megan still wasn't eating or drinking and my husband and I were desperately worried by this time. Her core temperature had plummeted but they didn't give her a blanket. And, again, they didn't give her any food or drink. However they did check her over for bruising…

Throughout I felt as if they were pointing the finger at her dad and me as the "cause" of Megan's apparent self-imposed starvation and distressed mental state. Goodness only knows what they thought we'd done to our daughter. It was horrible; truly horrible.

The nurse therapist from CAMHS came into the hospital to see us. I asked her for advice but she simply said that it wasn't her place to offer advice. So that was it, really.

A couple of weeks before, when I hadn't been able to sleep, I was desperately searching online for help at 3am. I followed link after link after link until I eventually came across the F.E.A.S.T. website and its forum, Around The Dinner Table which offers support to parents of young people with eating disorders. It was a lifesaver at a time when we didn't seem to be getting much support from anywhere else. For the first time I felt I was with a group of other parents who understood what we were going through.

Meanwhile, Megan was admitted to a residential adolescent mental health unit about two or three hours' drive away from our home. She was there for about three-and-a-half weeks. During this time she scarcely ate or drank a thing. We went in to see her every day and on one occasion I remember being so desperate to get her to eat that I sat there holding half a cereal bar. I said: "Megan, I love you, but if you don't eat this then I am going to have to walk out because I just can't bear to see you like this."

She ate it - all 35 calories of it.

Meanwhile her weight continued to drop. By the time we got her back home she was eating no more than 100 or 150 calories a day. But at least she was away from the unit and safely back at home. Now her dad and I could focus on doing the real work, the work that the professionals should have been doing: getting Megan to eat and drink again, and getting her well.

It was horrendous, it really was. Megan became violent and irrational. It was terrifying and it was heart-breaking. Initially our hopes were raised a little when we heard about a new eating disorders service in the area which offered support. Someone would come to our home for an hour a day. They were obviously kind and wanted to help. I assumed this would be to show us how to get Megan to eat successfully. But they didn't do this. Instead their new support workers seemed to be more interested in psychotherapy - in talking rather than "doing". It was upsetting for Megan; it was upsetting for all of us. We told them we felt it wasn't working so that was the end of that.

Okay, we thought, we've got no choice but to knuckle down and do this by ourselves. We had to get our daughter well and we knew that no-one else was going to do this for us. And at least our own knowledge on eating disorders was up to date. So we went back to all the reference books we'd bought earlier, and bought new ones, and worked out a plan.

We arranged to get Megan's weight and blood pressure checked out at the GPs' practice every couple of days, and every couple of months we'd visit a psychiatrist to assess her medication. Apart from this we just sat there and fed our daughter three meals and three snacks a day whether she wanted to eat or not. There was enormous resistance.

It was the toughest period of my life and I spent many, many a sleepless night listening to her howl, roar and scream for hours, holding her tight while she cried or to stop her from exercising and talking softly to distract her from the tortuous thoughts and feelings. For more than five months, she slept with me while my husband took up residence in the spare room, which meant broken nights for everyone.

One night I remember creeping into the spare room and saying to my husband: "So, we've got three or four months' re-feeding, a year's maintenance and a lifetime of vigilance." Without hesitation, we both said: "We can do that!" It wasn't going to be easy, but we'd do it, no matter what the illness threw at us.

So we battled on with the re-feeding. On one particular occasion, when we were trying to get Megan to eat a snack, we hit another complete refusal to eat and drink. She stood there sobbing and screaming for a full two hours, punching and kicking with her mouth and eyes shut, shouting: "I can't! I tried! I just can't do it anymore!" Food and vitriol from the eating disorder were flying. Meanwhile I'd taken care to ensure her younger siblings were as far away from the commotion as possible, in the furthest bedroom with the music on, so as not to upset them.

We calmly went through what would happen if Megan didn't eat: doctor, hospital, possibly being tube-fed... We offered to replace the snack with a shake, but she still refused. There was no-one I could call for assistance, so I posted up an urgent cry for help on the ATDT forum. One of the UK members immediately emailed me with her phone number even though it was Sunday morning. I just sat there and sobbed while she calmed me down, offered me advice and told me what she used to do in this kind of situation. I came back downstairs with calm resolve and told Megan that I knew she could do it; my strength was right there for her and so was her dad's.

Later I asked Megan what had caused the outburst. She said she'd caught a reflection of herself in a window (we'd hidden the mirrors months ago) and hated herself. She said she'd never get better; she just wanted to die. I calmly explained that we would never let her die, that we loved her and that she was too wonderful, compassionate and creative to lose. So whether we did it at home, in hospital or through a tube, we would ensure she got the nutrition she needed to get well. We told her that we loved her and had missed her, so we'd far rather do it at home. Later she did eat successfully and then we all went out together. It was exhausting, but I had my sights set on full recovery for my daughter, regardless of what it took.

Gradually, over time, Megan began to put on weight and - with the help of the books, the forum, our own sheer hard work and Megan's emerging determination to recover from this terrifying illness - we slowly but surely got her back to her pre-eating disorder weight. She returned to school and now, in the spring of 2013, she's just about to sit for her GCSE examinations.

Megan has been weight restored for nearly two years and it's now five months since she last self-harmed, something which she would do regularly at the height of her eating disorder.

She looks just like any other normal teenage girl. But underneath there are still some residual issues. For instance she insists on wearing baggy clothes. Also, she's very much of an avoider and still suffers from anxiety - and she won't talk to anyone about her worries or feelings.

But the good news is that her weight is fine and she's eating okay. She still hasn't cottoned onto the idea that *she* needs to eat, even when her friends *aren't* eating. Also, she went on a sleepover a couple of weeks ago and we had to bump the weight back up afterwards. But on the whole she's fine. She's a gorgeous girl, and it's all down to us working together as a strong family team.

But, as I said at the beginning, our story could have had a very different ending. For a start, I'd read up on eating disorders so I knew what we were dealing with and what needed to be done. Also, as a teacher, I was already aware of CAMHS. But what if I'd never heard of them? What if we'd never read all those books?

In our own personal experience, clinicians' understanding of eating disorders - or lack of understanding - is shocking. I'm not talking about layman's understanding where you read up on eating disorders like we did, but proper grassroots training on the latest evidence-based treatment for, and research into, eating disorders.

For example we saw a psychiatrist at one point along the line who diagnosed Megan as being "depressed". We said, "Well of course she's depressed; she's got an eating disorder". But it didn't seem to register. Also, we had a big set-to about the fact that she was on this 50th centile and CAMHS said her weight was fine. I remember sitting in front of this psychiatrist as he kept pointing at the 50th centile on a graph explaining what being in the 50th centile meant. I thought: "I'm an intelligent person. *I know* what a 50th centile is. But I also know that it's not right for my daughter." So I told him that Megan had always been in the 85th centile, ever since she was a toddler, so why on earth would she need to be anything other than that now? He agreed to disagree, choosing to overlook the fact that she'd just lost three stone in as many months.

Another thing… the whole falling off a cliff business happened so horribly quickly. Initially the descent into the eating disorder was so gradual we scarcely noticed anything. Then she suddenly lost five pounds and it was like - whallop! - the eating disorder had her in its grip. Suddenly she was throwing up. Suddenly she was pulling her hair out, screaming and getting violent. It happened so very quickly; it was horrifying.

At one point we saw a psychologist who said, "But she's very young to be developing an eating disorder".

I said: "No, she isn't. She's almost 14 and that's the average age that young people develop eating disorders." I immediately thought: "What exactly do these professionals know?"

As a schoolteacher I am under constant pressure to keep up to speed with the latest research, curriculum changes and so on. I am expected to keep my knowledge base completely up to date.

So our experience with health professionals both puzzles and disturbs me. Eating disorders are the biggest killer of all mental health disorders, yet there we were, forced to care for our own daughter without appropriate, educated support because the professionals simply weren't equipped to do the job.

Another thing that still shocks me is this…

I've already talked about A&E checking for bruising. But there were other occasions, too, when the finger was being clearly pointed at us, the parents. It was as if they were saying: "What did you do to cause the eating disorder?"

I'm the breadwinner in our family and so it was my husband who took Megan along to the GPs' surgery for regular check-ups when we were re-feeding her. Sometimes the nurse would say to Megan, "It's okay, your dad doesn't have to come into the room with you" and once she'd closed the door she'd ask if there was anything Megan would like to tell her now that her dad wasn't present.

It was horrendous. It was awful. The automatic assumption that it's the parents who are at fault; indeed the implication that we - a normal, happy, loving family - could be abusing our beautiful daughter was truly horrible.

If it was any other life-threatening illness like cancer or a heart condition, no-one in their right minds would blame the parents, let alone suspect abuse. Nor would clinicians be so dangerously uninformed about the serious condition they were responsible for treating.

There would be uproar.

MY TIPS:

Get educated. Buy books and join F.E.A.S.T. and its forum ATDT (see list of resources at the end of this book).

Treat your child with compassion. The eating disorder is not their fault; it is not a lifestyle choice, it is a biological brain disorder.

Be assertive with the professionals. Insist on being present at all meetings with your child (preferably without your child initially) until you are completely confident that the professionals know what they're doing. Check out the F.E.A.S.T. for a wealth of information.

Paul's & Jayne's story

"Eleanor took the information she picked up from appearing on Channel 4's *Supersize vs Superskinny* and, by sheer willpower, applied it to herself. She refused to give in to the illness."

Paul: Eleanor was 13 when I first met her. I was 15. Initially we were "just friends", but by the time Eleanor was 15 it had blossomed into a proper relationship. Eleanor was always happy, confident and bubbly, which is one of the many things that attracted me to her. I proposed to her on her 18th birthday in October 2005 and she said "Yes!" However we were both keen for her to finish her studies at college before getting married. We bought our first house together in July 2007 and married one year later in August 2008.

Jayne: Eleanor is our only child. She'd always had a sunny and outgoing personality. In fact she was just a normal teenager with a small but close circle of friends. She was also very bright, always getting great school reports for effort and behaviour. Eleanor never had any problems with food, either. She had a great appetite and would eat whatever I put in front of her. Basically, there were no problems at all before the anorexia struck.

Paul: Looking back, things started to change in early 2007 when Eleanor was 19, just before we bought our first house together.

Jayne: We used to love to sit in the kitchen together over a cuppa and a snack. On one occasion I was making toast and offered her a slice. Well, she practically bit my head off. But it was the tone of her voice that made my blood run cold; a tone so unlike Eleanor's "real" voice that it was almost unrecognisable. "I don't want to eat, leave me alone!" she yelled in this frightening new tone. It may sound crazy but it was almost as if she were "possessed" or completely consumed by "something". It was enough to terrify me. What in heaven's name was happening to my beautiful, happy, friendly daughter - the girl I'd always been so very close to?

Paul: I noticed that Eleanor was becoming more distant and quiet. She was getting quite moody. For example in early 2007 we went away with my family to Cornwall and Eleanor didn't speak to anyone all week. I also noticed that she was becoming obsessive about things as well as indecisive and generally unhappy. It as if she'd lost her sparkle and her sense of humour. In fact her emotions seemed to be pretty much flat-lining with very little variation. Meanwhile she hardly had a word to say to any of us and this wasn't like Eleanor, it really wasn't. I remember her saying that she felt so alone even though she was with all of us.

Even the task of getting up and dressed in the morning became a challenge. Eleanor would try on numerous outfits, constantly changing her mind. This could take anything up to an hour and I remember the bedroom being littered with crumpled dresses, jeans, tee-shirts, tops and shoes. And you could bet your back teeth that whatever outfit she'd eventually decide on wouldn't be "right".

One day a friend and I went to get our hair cut while Eleanor went shopping with my cousin. In a shoe shop she found herself in front of a wall of shoes - all similar styles but in three different colours. My cousin was alarmed at what happened next. It was almost as though Eleanor had a breakdown over which pair to choose. She'd frantically pick up each colour and try them on, one by one, giving my cousin a rapid summary of what she thought about each shoe and why she liked them - or didn't. Then she'd go through them all again.

"What about these? These will go with any colour. But, no, I prefer this pair... What do you think about these? No, I'm not sure... Will they match these trousers? Or any trousers? What about with a skirt?"

On and on and on it went at a million miles an hour like some kind of nightmarish stuck record. She just couldn't choose. No, it was more serious than that, she had lost the *ability* to choose.

Jayne: Eleanor was still living at home at this point. We'd always eaten our meals together. It was a great opportunity talk about what kind of day we'd had. If she was going out with Paul, going dancing or rehearsing a show, then it would be a bit of a rush tea. But we still insisted on eating together. I did the cooking and made sure meals were always on the table ready for when Eleanor returned from school or college, and my husband Tony got back from work.

But suddenly Eleanor began insisting on taking her meal up to her room. She wouldn't eat with her dad and me. She *was* eating. Or at least she was eating *most* of it. She just couldn't face being watched while she ate.

When she moved in with Paul I didn't see her for a couple of weeks. Then one weekend Paul was away and I drove over to keep Eleanor company. We'd arranged to go shopping and I remember Eleanor coming down the stairs, dressed and ready to go. My heart did a nose dive. The clothes that had always fitted her snugly were just hanging off her. Indeed she was having a battle to keep her trousers from falling down her hips. It was at this point that I began to seriously wonder if we had a problem on our hands. I'd never seen her as slim as this.

Paul: Before she got sick, Eleanor and I would often go out for meals. Or, if we were in town, we'd pop into MacDonald's and pick up a burger, that kind of thing. Just like normal people. But suddenly she wasn't interested anymore. I'd ask her what she'd like to eat and she'd just say: "Nothing, thanks." She wasn't aggressive or anything;

she was quite calm. I'd try to tempt her with items from the menu but she'd just say she was fine; she wasn't hungry.

Of course I had no idea what was happening to her. I did wonder whether she was trying to lose weight in order to get noticed by talent agencies. Eleanor is a stunning young woman and she was busy doing the rounds of modelling and acting agents.

Then, when the mood swings started, I thought it was directed at me; I thought I'd done something wrong. I was sad and confused. We'd just bought our first house together. It was something we'd been planning for ages and it should have been a happy, exciting occasion, but it wasn't, it was horrible. To be honest I got angry and began to worry if I'd done the right thing in moving in with her. I had no idea what was wrong.

Jayne: We had no idea what it was, either. You don't expect your child to get an eating disorder especially someone like Eleanor who'd always been healthy, happy and had eaten well. In my mind, eating disorders were something that happened to other families. A friend's daughter who is a few years younger than Eleanor had gone through anorexia. Her mum used to speak to me a lot; she used to get so stressed and upset about it. I'll never forget the day we visited my friend and saw her daughter. It was the day before this girl was admitted to an eating disorder unit. Her weight had plummeted since we last saw her. She was painfully thin. We also noticed that her lips were dry and flaking.

Apparently this girl had been bullied. Other girls had been calling her names and making cruel comments about her weight. Her mother was sure this had triggered the eating disorder. When we left the house Eleanor insisted she'd never let herself "get like that". And, because there was no obvious reason why my daughter would ever develop an eating disorder, I remember feeling relief; it wasn't going to happen to us.

How wrong I was.

Now, looking back, I often wonder what it was that triggered

Eleanor's anorexia. Unlike my friend's daughter, Eleanor had never been bullied. Maybe it was all the talk of dieting that girls go through at school and college. Or, I used to wonder, was she unhappy at home? There was no reason why she *would* be unhappy; we'd always been a very close family. The thing is, when someone changes like this, you do begin to puzzle over it.

One afternoon Eleanor and I went out for a drink. She'd taken the day off work and wanted a mother-and-daughter catch-up now she was living with Paul. We sat over our coffees for a couple of hours. In that time she poured it all out to me - everything she had been feeling and going through since January. She explained how confused she was. She described how she felt and what she was doing: how she was counting calories, weighing herself frequently, feeling depressed, lost and very, very unhappy.

I was alarmed when she said that she had "voices in her head" which would torment her after she'd eaten or whenever she looked in the mirror. It was as if they were yelling: "You greedy pig! You're worthless." These "voices" would push her and punish her by forcing her to exercise after eating. Sometimes she was so desperate to block out these voices that I would catch her clinging onto the arm of the sofa with her finger nails to stop "them" from making her stand up, get onto the floor and start a session of press-ups or sit-ups. Or I'd catch her clinging onto something heavy or fixed to the wall to prevent herself from exercising. It was as if she were being compelled to exercise against her will. These "voices" were her own personal bully.

Paul: I was confused and very, very worried. I still wondered if it was me - had I done something wrong? Had she fallen out of love with me? I felt upset and angry at the changes I was seeing in the girl I'd known so very well and for so long.

Jayne: Eleanor didn't seem to want to talk about it. So I kept quiet. I guess I just hoped it would go away of its own accord. But I must admit I was scared at what I was seeing. And because she wasn't talking to me about it, I felt incredibly helpless. Meanwhile Eleanor's unusual eating continued. She was also losing more weight. Gradually I began to realise what we were dealing with. The daughter of the friend had begun her treatment for anorexia. We compared notes and I put two and two together.

Paul: In July, prompted by her best friend and my cousin who were both worried, Eleanor went to see the GP who confirmed it was an eating disorder. I remember her coming back from the appointment. The whole family was there. It was a very emotional moment.

She walked in the door and told us everything that had gone on. The GP had diagnosed anorexia nervosa. So now it was "on paper", in "black and white": Eleanor had anorexia.

Well, her mum burst into tears. I just sat there open-mouthed while her dad kept quiet. I think he was worried sick. Then Eleanor broke down. She was in pieces. She almost didn't believe it herself. I remember her saying that, as she looked down at the diagnosis on paper, she saw nothing but an image of skull and crossbones, like on a toxic label. She felt that this was it. This illness would kill her. She was terrified.

Jayne: In a way it was good that Eleanor took it upon herself to visit the GP. By now her BMI was pretty low and I know she told the GP about her obsessive behaviours around food and weight. For example how she would count calories on labels, swap things for lower calorie options and weigh herself after every meal. But despite diagnosing Eleanor with anorexia, the GP seemed reluctant to get too involved, simply handing her some leaflets, giving her the contact details of a local eating disorders clinic and suggesting she come back every two to three weeks to get her weight checked. And that was all.

Because Eleanor was 18, we, as parents, weren't permitted any direct contact with the GP unless Eleanor gave her permission. But the impression we were getting was that the surgery didn't offer any particular support to patients with eating disorders.

Paul: The following January, Eleanor and I were watching TV together. It was the first series of Channel 4's *Supersize vs Superskinny*. Eleanor decided she needed a weight-gain food plan like the ones they were using on the diet swaps, so she emailed the producers for advice. But, instead of sending her a food plan, she got a phone call from Channel 4 asking her if she'd like to take part in the second series which was to feature a section about people suffering from eating disorders. Eleanor said yes. Filming was to begin in September, after our wedding.

Jayne: Meanwhile Eleanor agreed to seek professional help for her eating disorder. At first the GP was a little reluctant to offer counselling. But Eleanor pushed for it and got it. I attended the first session with her. In 60 minutes she poured out her heart. She broke down, saying how she felt so lost and had no idea where she was heading. She described her obsession with calories and restricted eating. She felt as though everything in her life was out of her control.

Eleanor attended a follow-up session with the counsellor, this time alone. Following this, she felt able to cope on her own and decided that no further sessions were required. Of course this was the eating disorder tricking everyone into thinking that she was just fine. It even had Eleanor fooled.

Much later she would tell me that, at the initial counselling session, she felt that the eating disorder was "another side" of her; a little person - a "demon" type thing - that controlled her. She felt as if she were dragging it kicking and screaming to that first appointment. But it was hell bent on keeping her within its clutches; it wasn't going to let go without a fight. At the second session Eleanor really felt that she'd got it under control when in fact, underneath, it was the "demon" that was dragging Eleanor kicking and screaming over the abyss. Little did any of us realise that, far from being in control, Eleanor was being dragged under fast.

Paul: Things were quite up and down for ages. We'd take a step forward only to be followed by a couple of steps back. I was aware that she was finding it a real struggle. By our wedding she was seriously worried that she might never recover.

To help her on a bit, and with the help of her mum, the staff in the wedding shop said that she could have the dress she wanted, but only on condition that she put on some weight. They refused to make any alterations. It was that particular size or nothing.

To be honest, I think this was the pivotal moment - the moment when Eleanor began to get the upper hand over the eating disorder. She worked like a Trojan to ensure that the wedding dress would fit by our wedding day. And I am thrilled to say she did it.

All husbands remember their wedding day. But, for me, I find it hard to describe how proud I felt of that beautiful young woman who walked up the aisle and stood next to me by the altar. Best of all, Eleanor was smiling - a stunning, happy smile that will stay with me forever.

It would be wrong of me to claim it was a miracle. Part of me was well aware that Eleanor still had some way to go. Just because she'd managed to put on enough weight to get into that wedding dress didn't mean she was free of the eating disorder. On our wedding day she only ate breakfast. And, anxious about being watched by all the guests as she sat at the top table, she didn't eat at the reception.

On our honeymoon she only ate small amounts. Then on the final day we went out to a restaurant. My heart sank when she looked at the menu and announced that she'd go without and wait until the in-flight meal that evening. Of course I didn't want to sit there eating alone, so when the waiter came over to take our order we made our excuses and left.

But there were some times when she would eat relatively normally. In fact I was quite impressed on one occasion when she ate her way through a two-course meal. To most people this might not seem like a lot, but when you're getting over an eating disorder it's a milestone. At the time I felt she was determined not to let the eating disorder spoil our honeymoon. Also, because her stomach was unused to large amounts of food, she began to experience stomach pains. Sometimes they were so acute that she'd double-up in pain, in tears, barely able to walk back to the hotel.

This scared her. It scared me, too. In fact I broke down. Neither of us had any idea what was happening and we both thought the worst. I thought: "This is it, if the anorexia didn't kill her before then it's going to kill her now, on our honeymoon."

But, in the event, it was just that her body wasn't used to food. She'd cut back so much that it would take time to get it used to normal portion sizes and regular eating.

Meanwhile filming for *Supersize vs Superskinny* began in September. The programme involved filming for one day a week for around eight weeks, taking part in tasks that would prove challenging for people with eating disorders, supported by a specialist eating disorders dietician and a couple of one-to-one sessions with an eating disorders specialist. Each filming session was followed by a 50-minute private consultant with a psychotherapist.

Ursula Philpot (*Supersize vs Superskinny* on screen dietician & Senior Lecturer at Leeds Metropolitan University's School of Health & Wellbeing, Advanced Practice Dietician and Mental Health Group Education Officer for the British Dietetic Association): It was a highly intensive eight weeks for everyone. Initially Eleanor and the others were individually assessed by a specialist psychotherapist, psychiatrist and myself. Then each week we'd focus on a different practical activity, usually revolving around food or social situations, depending on what the participants felt would be the most helpful.

For example we would look at meal planning and discuss particular challenges they were going to set themselves that week. We also did other activities which weren't filmed, for example helping them to tackle patterns of negative thinking and become more compassionate around themselves.

One therapeutic aspect which came about almost by accident was the fact that, in order to participate in the making of the programme, participants needed to get out of the house, get on a train and do other things that maybe they didn't feel too comfortable with. There was also a lot of interaction with the film crew, many of whom were of a similar age - so they were obliged to interact with them in a normal sociable setting, often involving meals. So all of this helped.

We didn't take over from the participants' regular clinicians; instead we worked very closely with them throughout. Not all the clinicians were willing to engage with us, however, but it's interesting that the most successful outcomes were those where the clinicians were happy to do this.

Paul: Of course, following the show, recovery wasn't instant by any means. Between that first visit to the GP and strong signs of recovery I would say it took approximately three years. Eleanor took the information she'd picked up from the TV programme and, by sheer willpower, applied it to herself. More than anything Eleanor wanted to have a baby and she knew that, until she got her weight up, this wasn't going to happen. For a start, she hadn't had a period for over eighteen months. She was also keen to recover from the anorexia before she gave birth. She didn't want to be an anorexic mum. She didn't want her health issues to affect her child in any way.

In May 2009 Eleanor discovered she was pregnant. We saw this as a miracle baby! Our son was born on 1st January 2010 weighing a healthy 7 pounds 13 oz. Two years later in April 2012 he was followed by a brother - another healthy baby, the babies we might never have had if Eleanor's eating disorder had taken a turn for the worse.

Eleanor is now 25 and we're just like any other normal family with two growing boys. The eating disorder is well and truly gone and we're looking forward to a great future together. I'd like to pay tribute to Eleanor for her strength, courage and determination to refuse to let the anorexia win. Recovery can't have been easy for her; I know because I was with her most of the time, but she was determined to get well. And she succeeded.

Jayne: Looking back, Eleanor's anorexia was a really tough time for everyone. As a young couple, planning to buy a house, get married and start a family, eating together is a normal part of life. But Eleanor and Paul simply couldn't do this because of the illness. While Eleanor was still living at home, she'd insist on the same menu, week in, week out, because she found it so very hard to eat. She developed obsessions about certain foods. For instance on Tuesdays she allowed herself to eat cheese twists. But they always had to be from the same bakery, and only on Tuesdays, never any other day. If we got there and they'd sold out, it was sheer panic and we'd have to dash around to try and find another branch of the same bakery, selling the same item, because if we didn't then it would tip the balance and Eleanor would refuse to eat anything else. I'd far rather she ate the cheese twists than nothing!

As her parents, we got no help or support from the health services. It was Eleanor's sheer determination to beat the illness that kept us going, really. She has recovered with the help of others but first and foremost through her own strength and determination. She has raised and brought two beautiful grandchildren into the world. Nowadays she uses her knowledge and experience to help others and raise awareness of eating disorders.

As a mother, my advice would be to keep a careful watch for unusual behaviour and be sure to contact organisations like Beat (the UK eating disorders charity), ABC (Anorexia & Bulimia Care) and F.E.A.S.T. for advice and support. The internet is a great source of information for this kind of thing, especially online forums like Around The Dinner Table for parents of young people with eating disorders.

Amanda's story

"'Just how far will you go?' I asked my daughter. 'There is no end,' she said. Terrified, I promised her there and then that, whether she hated me for the rest of her life, I was fighting for her very survival."

It's odd how you remember conversations you had with your children that meant "nothing" at the time but, in hindsight, you realise how important they were. Those moments when they ask: "Is it you?" meaning are we Father Christmas? And those moments when your beautiful, perfect and, to all intents and purposes, normal daughter begins to talk about body shape and pointing out how some jeans are made for different shapes than others.

The first time my - then - 15-year old daughter, Ellie, and I had one of these conversations I remember thinking: "That was weirdly out of proportion." It was during the Easter holiday of 2009 and Ellie was talking about the prospect of a summer holiday with some friends. These friends have three daughters who grew like beanpoles. At the time Ellie was about a foot shorter than the eldest. Her reaction was really extreme. It went something along the lines of: "Well, I won't go on holiday with them. There's no way I could lie next to T--- by the pool 'cause I'm just so huge!"

I was horrified that she thought this way about herself, but brushed it over with a loving response of somewhere between "there, there" and "don't be so silly". In the event, and for reasons totally unrelated to that, the holiday never took place.

A couple of months later, Ellie took four of her GCSE

examinations early; she was one of the brighter pupils in her year group. It was then that I noticed she was self-harming - nothing too dramatic, just scratching herself and not allowing it to heal. But it was enough to make me notice and assume the exams must be causing her stress. Then in August when the results came out, one of them was a B. Forget about the fact that the other three were As; Ellie saw the B as "failure", so much so that she couldn't celebrate the success.

During that summer Ellie made an attempt to diet, just to shift a couple of pounds. To me this was normal teenage behaviour, so I wasn't unduly concerned. The diet didn't work, so she stopped. It didn't really cross my radar. Perhaps it should have done. In the autumn I remember asking a friend (with older daughters) how one talks about these things with teenage girls. By then something must have worried me enough to ask a question like this. Then I went away for a week. Meanwhile Ellie developed a virus which meant she couldn't eat.

That's when I believe "it" got in.

On my return, Ellie talked of having lost four pounds. She also said her periods were a "bit weird". I remember brushing it off with a "don't worry you'll soon be back to normal" comment.

Meal times started to get fraught. She'd leave food untouched and refuse some food types. I remember getting very angry over a baked potato and some gammon. Actually I was so cross that I mentally took a step back from the situation and thought "this line of attack isn't working; I need to think how to get round this in a better way". I tried cajoling and cooking her favourite foods. I asked what she had eaten at lunch thinking that if she'd eaten a good school lunch then I needn't be so worried about what she wasn't eating at home.

I was beginning to lose sleep over it. Ellie was beginning to lie about what she was eating at school. I knew this because she talked about eating cottage pie and she never ate cottage pie at school! Her breakfast became a pint of black coffee and an apple. When her younger brother reported that she was having the same for school lunch, I knew something was wrong. The tension in the house was beginning to rise around meal times. I began to be thrilled if I saw anything edible pass her lips. But more than once I thought: "It can't be anorexia because anorexics don't eat anything at all."

I noticed that Ellie was finding it hard to keep warm. Chilblains set in that actually made her cry. She said she thought her toes were going to fall off. Worried, I had a chat with one of her friends who told me how concerned she was about Ellie. I'm a nurse by profession and immediately I put on my nurse's hat, so to speak, and began to think about anorexia. That afternoon I confronted my daughter. It didn't go well and the shutters came down. But the gloves were off. I had thrown the "anorexia word" into the conversation and told her how fearful and worried we all were. I asked where the money I gave her for school lunches was. Two hours later a shoe box with two months' worth of school dinner money was handed to me.

Initially I thought: "This can't be happening to us." Ellie was always such a good girl. She was always highly thought of and had always been taught not to lie. She was well behaved at school, was very popular and had boyfriends. We were hugely proud of her in every way.

We are just a normal, close, "functioning" family; there is nothing unusual about us. If anything, we're the kind of family that, to others, might appear to "have it all". But, as time went on, that couldn't have been less true. With the arrival of an "unwanted extra" in our midst, we became a dysfunctional family. We didn't change immediately; we were still the five of us, going about our daily lives. But, to the professionals, we became dysfunctional.

I rang the GP. She rang me back right away and I sobbed Ellie's story to her down the phone while she listened patiently. The GP acted fast and told me to bring Ellie in under the pretext of the chilblains and let her do the rest.

We arrived and I was allowed into the consultation where the GP asked Ellie some gentle, quiet and insightful questions. Was she feeling okay? Was she a bit stressed? Had she noticed losing weight?

Ellie admitted to losing a stone so far, but she insisted she was okay and that there was nothing to worry about. But the GP *was* worried. She asked us to return in two weeks for another weigh-in and chat. If she saw deterioration then Ellie would be referred to CAMHS. It was Christmas 2009.

Two weeks later and another four pounds lighter, Ellie begged for more time so she could stop losing weight. The GP gave her a week. I started to leak (cry) a lot. Surely the 500 calories a day she was eating wasn't enough to stop the weight loss?

Back at school, the horror texts started with messages about how she couldn't cope with everyone looking at her, how she wasn't good enough to be liked or loved. She lost another four pounds.

Thankfully the CAMHS referral came very quickly. Our first appointment was with a nurse at the local child and family mental health unit. Ellie was furious. She refused to talk. The nurse asked patronising questions like: "Is this your mum? What's her name?" I was sitting right there! And "Is this your dad? What's his name?" Ellie sat tight lipped while I fumed. I mean, Ellie was an intelligent articulate 15-year old girl, not a four year old child in need of cajoling. So, to be honest, I wasn't surprised when Ellie refused to go back. However, we persisted for a while. The patronising tone continued and Ellie continued to not eat. She was two stone down by now. An emergency psychiatrist was called in for an assessment; we needed a diagnosis for our skiing holiday insurance. Well, we just needed a diagnosis, full stop. The usual psychiatrist was on holiday.

The GP and the emergency psychiatrist were exemplary in their thoughtful, insightful and trust-inducing help in a situation that was fast spinning out of control with no apparent brakes in sight.

The emergency psychiatrist talked about how we shouldn't trust anything Ellie might say to us about food and that she couldn't be relied on to be telling the truth. She talked about food being Ellie's medicine and insisted we increase her calories and give her six meals a day - three main meals and three snacks. We were to go home and feed her on hot buttered toast and hot chocolate. At last I had instructions. I naïvely thought to myself, yes, I can feed my child with this kind of stuff. After all, how hard could it be?

We were in a town a couple of hours from home. The café was crowded. I placed the toast and hot chocolate in front of Ellie while she stared at it as if I'd offered her poison. She picked at it, eating the tiniest mouthfuls and cried. She didn't finish it. From what she told me years later she kept it in her mouth and spat it out in the car. But at the time I had no idea that this kind of thing could happen. I was just so horrified at how, when I fed my daughter food, the "monster" reared its ugly head and fought back. I am grateful that no-one in that café knew us.

I went from being the happy, chatty mother at mealtimes to being my daughter's gaoler. Or at least that's how it felt. I became savvy at watching as surreptitiously as possible at mealtimes, open-mouthed at the "monster's" wily tricks of stashing food up sleeves, throwing things around, smashing stuff and running out of the room.

Desperate to find out more about what was consuming my daughter, I began to read. Book after book after book. I equipped myself with Lock and Le Grange's *Help Your Teenager Beat An Eating Disorder* (another nugget from the emergency psychiatrist). I also became familiar with Janet Treasure's *Skills-Based Learning for Caring for a Loved One with an Eating Disorder* and learned about her animal metaphors for different types of carer.

I was very quickly realising that Ellie needed me to fight for her survival. Yet at the same time I was falling apart, silently weeping and mourning the loss of my dear daughter who had changed beyond recognition, mentally and physically. The "real" Ellie had completely disappeared, just like her weight. Of course our, then, eight year old youngest son didn't understand what was happening. "I just want my Ellie back," he whispered to me one morning.

Meanwhile, we saw CAMHS weekly. Ellie was also weighed at the GPs' surgery. By now we were seeing the regular psychiatrist again. At the very first meeting she told us that Ellie wasn't thin enough to be diagnosed with anorexia. Now, I am not a swearing woman, but -

boy - did I swear then! "I'm not bl***y standing around waiting for her to get thin enough!" I shouted at her.

Of course Ellie - or rather the "monster" that had replaced Ellie - saw this as a triumph and "official permission" to carry on losing weight... three stone in as many months by this time.

Every week the psychiatrist would ask her how she was feeling. On those weeks when the GP couldn't see her, I remember the psychiatrist telling Ellie that she "looked like she was gaining weight". The result of these less-than-artful comments? Hours of self-harming, berating and loathing once we got home.

Ellie couldn't sleep. I didn't sleep. I would sit on her bed, stroking her back for hours on end, willing her to realise that she was loved and willing her to eat. I'd tell her stories of her childhood, remembering happier times. Praying. Hoping. Losing hope and losing time.

Gradually I realised that I had to be strong. I had to fight on Ellie's behalf against the eating disorder. I couldn't just sit there, go to pieces and leak my way through umpteen boxes of Kleenex tissues. I'd always been the strong one. I'd always known what to do. Now I had to be strong. I had to fight. I had no choice.

By this time Ellie couldn't face school. One day she begged me to pick her up. She couldn't face lunchtimes. She couldn't face her friends seeing how "hideously fat" she was. All I was seeing was a girl who was losing weight fast, who was developing the tell-tale peardrops smell on her breath, had a vacant look in her eyes and a dreadful pallor that made her skin almost translucent. Her frozen fingers, toes and expression... All were lost to the illness that consumed her mind and thoughts.

We removed Ellie from school. She didn't return for nine months. Her GCSEs became unimportant, unattainable. They could wait.

I realised that, although I was never "pushy" (having failed all my school exams I never expected my kids to be brilliant), I did have dreams for my kids' futures. Who doesn't? But, at this time, I began to reassess these dreams. I wondered if Ellie would ever have relationships again. Her friends had stopped visiting and she hated herself. I wondered if she'd ever go out again. She was just too scared to be seen in public.

I grieved. Yes, that's what I did in those months… I grieved and I fought. But I fought the illness, not Ellie. I fought for her existence. I even rang the Government demanding a specialist dietician for our area. It was provided but only for Adult Services.

I rang various advocacy groups. Surely my daughter needed specialist help? Going to CAMHS didn't seem to be doing anything. It was a bit like taking your child to see the GP over and over again with a broken leg when really she needed to see an orthopaedic surgeon. CAMHS didn't seem to "get it". And I felt judged not supported. Meanwhile I continued to read anything I could get my hands on about eating disorders. I read avidly morning, noon and night. Well, mostly during the night as sleeping became impossible.

Our happy, close, normal family because a statistic: a dysfunctional family. Our marriage was crumbling, our daughter was dying and our two sons were floundering around without the normality of our "old" life.

By the summer of 2010 Ellie's weight had stabilised. She wasn't losing as fast and we had worked so hard on trust. She was now managing to eat what I put in front of her. Okay, it still wasn't enough and there was still a lot of food that she wouldn't touch. But at least she wasn't running out of the house into the snow with only her pjs on, getting lost for hours while friends and family combed the fields looking for her. She was able to eat in front of the TV and, occasionally, at the table with the family. I saw all of these things as small steps in the right direction.

By now I'd found a superb online resource called F.E.A.S.T. and its forum, Around The Dinner Table, for parents of young people with eating disorders. Through these two resources I learned an enormous amount. I also continued to read. And you know what? Everything I was discovering pointed towards the fact that my child must eat to recover. Now, to the uninitiated, that might sound obvious. Starving people need to eat. But, strangely, not once had CAMHS (bar the emergency psychiatrist at the beginning) mentioned that Ellie needed to eat to get well.

So, as a family, we made a radical decision. We quit CAHMS and moved Ellie's treatment to a specialist private eating disorder unit two hours' drive from our home. Initially we attended twice a week. The first time Ellie went there she came out smiling, exclaiming: "They understand, mum!"

They had talked to her about the fine hair on her body, her lack of periods and the need to eat. They had congratulated her on her triumphs thus far in halting the tumble downwards and they began to work with her. In just two hours they had gained her trust - and ours. They also cost my parents and in-laws a small fortune...

My husband and I were kept out of the loop apart from a few ten-minute sessions at the end to ask how things were going from our perspective. I found myself between a rock and a hard place. If I told them how it *really* was I'd have two hours of sulking and trying to jump from the car on the journey home. (No, not me, Ellie...) If I pretended everything was okay, then it wasn't so traumatic. So some days I pretended, other days I went greyer!

That September Ellie returned to school for the sixth form, initially part-time then gradually full-time. Bit by bit I began to see a blossoming of hope and signs of recovery. Her therapists had given her the tools to handle the stresses thrown at her. She was discharged after 18 months of treatment and, at first, I was delighted.

Sadly, though, unbeknown to me she had been discharged at a sub-optimal weight. Also, she wasn't given any follow-up with the result that she relapsed quite significantly while studying for her A-level examinations. I remember weeping to my mother on the phone: "I just can't go through this again, mum!"

"Yes you can," came the reply. So we did, but this time Ellie had the tools to see that real life was far more important and that the recovery she'd already glimpsed wasn't as far away as before. Gradually she cottoned on that, yes, life is worth living and that, with help and encouragement, she would make it back.

It is now April 2013 and Ellie is in a gap year before going to university. She is spending the year living away from home. Yes, she is thin. But I guess she might always be this way. She knows she can't ever "diet" again or even miss meals. She is well aware that the "ED voice" comes back if she doesn't have her snacks. She knows that it's still a bit of a knife-edge existence, but she also knows how to pull it back if the eating disorder comes knocking.

The professionals talk about independence with eating. They talk about families pulling back from treatment, not being so involved, especially with adult sufferers. My reply has always been that, although most good parents encourage their children to be independent, there are times when - if they fall, through illness or otherwise - it is still our responsibility to step in. And if that means "nursing" them back to a place where they can take that independence back, then that's what we'll do, regardless of their age.

I'll never forget the day I stood next to my, then, 15-year old daughter whilst she hugged the radiator through sheer cold because she just couldn't warm up - her fingers blue with cold, her skin pale and her breath smelling of peardrops, a vacant look in her eyes.

"Just how far will you go?" I asked her. "There is no end," she said. At that moment the fight for life took over and I promised her there and then that I would fight the illness that was "consuming" her every thought. I promised that, whether she hated me for the rest of her life, I was fighting for her very survival. I would know that as her mother I had and was doing the right thing, and hopefully one day she would thank me.

I couldn't stand by and watch my wonderful, gorgeous and in my eyes perfect daughter be killed by something too big for her to fight herself. As a family we encouraged and rooted for her, cheering her bravery and quietly loving the fact that she was on the road to health again, singing daily and able to go to parties, shop with friends and eat at the table with us. Now she is in recovery. At last we have a teenager who does teenager stuff. We so nearly didn't.

MY TIPS:

Get reading. Order these books: *Skills-Based Learning For Caring For A Loved One With An Eating Disorder: The New Maudsley Method* by Janet Treasure and *Help Your Teenager Beat an Eating Disorder* by David Lock & Daniel Le Grange. (See list of resources at the end of the book.)

Put yourself in your child's shoes. I was told to imagine that having an eating disorder (anorexia in our case) made food and the fear of getting fat the scariest thing ever, like being in a room full of spiders or snakes.

There is hope. Eating disorders, although extremely dangerous, are treatable through patience, persistence and love.

Food is medicine. I firmly believe that recovery starts at home. We are with our children most. We are the food providers. Food is their medicine.

Never go by look. It is a myth to believe that someone with an eating disorder needs to look emaciated.

Separate your child from the eating disorder. By separating the eating disordered thoughts and actions from your child, it gives strength to the "real" person that they are rather than the eating disorder.

Don't blame yourself. Your child's eating disorder is not your fault; it is a mental illness.

Take charge. Your child needs help and the security of knowing that adults who care and love them are there to fight on their behalf. Taking charge of eating when your child is unable to do so is imperative. Do not be afraid to do this. Get them to eat six times a day: three meals and three snacks i.e. breakfast, snack, lunch, snack, supper, snack.

Be patient, be consistent and be encouraging. It's tiring, it's difficult, it's lonely and it's tough but it's worth it!

Be vigilant. If there is a binge/purge element to the eating disorder (e.g. bulimia nervosa) take time following a meal to distract (games, TV, following them around the house and allowing no time alone) for at least an hour - to avoid purging.

Sadly an element of trust is lost to the disorder. It's hard to learn never to leave food and the eating disordered person alone. However, they will try to hide food or not eat. Be aware of this and always stay with them when they are eating. Unfortunately you can no longer believe that what they claim to have eaten has been eaten - unless you have seen it going in. Sadly this is a very deceptive illness, regardless of how honest and truthful the child was beforehand.

Find what works for you and your child. You have to decide what this is. Some people find that hiding calories (adding cream, butter, etc) works. Others find that trust, making a contract that nothing will be hidden, but that what is given must be eaten is another way of food introduction.

Gina's story

"I could see the consultant making notes, concluding that anxiety was the problem in the family and that our son was feeding off this atmosphere. Well of course we were anxious! What parents wouldn't be anxious?!"

If there's one thing that my young son, Adam, loved more than anything in the world it was going to visit family in Wales for a couple of weeks during the school summer holidays. We'd go there every single summer to visit my mum and dad - Adam's grandparents - and my sister who lived in the same village. It was one great big family gathering and everyone looked forward to it enormously. Better still, they all lived by the sea, so it was all about driving down there, dropping off the luggage and rushing down to the beach to mess around or do some rock pooling. Adam was in seventh heaven.

Then in the summer of 2011, when Adam was 10, everything changed. Things were different anyway because my mum and dad had both passed away a few months earlier. My husband, Colin, wasn't able to stay with us for the whole two weeks, due to work. But the plan was that he'd drive us to Wales, drop us off, go back to work and pick us up at the end of the fortnight.

It was while we were in Wales that I began to notice unusual things about Adam. Firstly, he seemed to be cold all the time. It was the height of summer and normally he'd be running around in shorts and tee-shirts, but instead he was wrapping himself up in fleeces, complaining of the cold.

He was getting upset for no obvious reason. I also noticed some slightly odd behaviour around food. Adam had always loved fruit. He'd eat fruit as if it was going out of fashion. But this particular summer he wouldn't touch it at all. I also remember my sister offering him some of her mother-in-law's wonderful home-made Bara Brith which he'd always loved, but he didn't want any. Then, oddly, I'd occasionally catch him coming back and grabbing something off the table when he thought no-one was looking. Yet he wouldn't accept food if it was offered to him. Also, unbeknown to any of us, he was doing a tremendous amount of exercise.

So there he was behaving strangely and getting upset when he was normally so happy in Wales. I just couldn't put my finger on it. I especially remember the day Colin returned to drive us all home. The first thing he did was offer to take all the kids down to the beach to do some rock pooling. Normally Adam would have jumped at that, but he just stood there and burst into tears. It was really odd. I remember we told Adam that he needed to eat or we'd have to take him to the doctor. But we really just left it at that. At the time he seemed to agree and said he would eat more. The idea that Adam might be developing an eating disorder never entered my mind. It doesn't when you have a boy, especially a boy as young as Adam.

Back home, Adam continued to act strangely. He was becoming even fussier over food, crying a great deal and his mood was pretty low much of the time. He used to enjoy playing with his sisters, but that all changed and he seemed to have no time for them anymore. He seemed to find them irritating.

It was the continued food avoidance that made me wonder whether he was developing an eating disorder. So, just before he went back to school in September, Colin and I went to see the GP. She was really brilliant and asked us all to come back a few days later for an extended appointment.

First the GP spoke to all of us and then she talked with Adam alone. She knew that eating disorders needed to be treated seriously and was more than happy to refer Adam to a specialist. She wrote us a "to whom it may concern" letter so we could claim for private treatment off the medical insurance that comes as part of my husband's work package.

Colin rang CAMHS to see if we could make an appointment to see their main consultant as private patients. But the consultant was on holiday, so the receptionist suggested we see CAMHS under the NHS. We actually got an appointment just two weeks later in the middle of September. So it all happened really quickly and from that point of view we were lucky. That was probably the last time we felt lucky for a very long time.

I'll always remember that first session with CAMHS. In a nutshell, they concluded that we were the neurotic parents and there was nothing wrong with Adam. The thing is, we knew he'd lost weight. But we had no idea what his start weight had been. Here in the UK children's weights aren't monitored after baby stage. Also, Adam had never been fat or skinny - he'd always seemed a normal, average weight to us. So, even though he had definitely lost some weight by this time, his weight was still falling within the "normal" range. So the alarm bells weren't ringing in the clinicians' heads.

Adam hardly spoke at all during the session. Colin did most of the talking. He tends to be very open. He's had anxiety issues of his own as well as a brief flirtation with disordered eating as a teenager. He mentioned all this to the CAMHS team who, after further probing into our past including the fact that we'd recently had a double bereavement in the family, concluded that *we* were the ones with the problem and that our son was perfectly fine. I could see the consultant making little notes, concluding that anxiety was the problem in the family and that our son was feeding off this atmosphere. Well of course we were anxious! Our son was behaving strangely, was losing weight and we were sitting in front of a team of mental health professionals. What parents wouldn't be anxious?!

I remember the consultant asking Adam what his plans were for after the session. Adam said we were going to MacDonald's. It was the worst thing he could have said, instantly confirming CAMHS' impression that everything was okay.

The thing is, Adam was still eating at this point, but not in the way he used to. This - along with the mood swings - is how we knew something was seriously wrong. However CAMHS asked us to come back in a few months' time, just so they could keep an eye on things.

Not very long ago I was talking to Adam about this period. He told me he'd felt really happy after the appointment - happy he'd been able to "hide behind us" as he put it. He'd "got away with it". And he really had!

Adam was ill, yet no-one could see this. But, because the professionals had given him a clean bill of health, we felt sure they must know best. Indeed I remember laughing with relief as we left CAMHS after that first appointment, joking to Adam that "Your parents are crazy, but you're fine!" We felt enormous relief. We thought everything was going to be alright. Remember, I knew nothing about anorexia at this stage; not one thing. But I do now!

If you were to ask me what I believe triggered Adam's emerging eating disorder I'd say that it was something that happened six months or so before that 2011 holiday in Wales. The Christmas before, my dad died of cancer. Then, just three months later, my mum passed away. As you can imagine, this period was incredibly stressful for the whole family. I was away a lot, visiting my dad in hospital in Wales before he died and then staying with my sister to help with funeral arrangements and so on.

Adam absolutely adored his grandparents. But, to be truthful, I was too wrapped up in my own grief to really notice how the rest of the family was handling it. It was a bit easier for my two daughters, because they were still so very young. But Adam took it very hard. The problem was I didn't know, because he hid it so well. I assumed he was coping really well, even though I'd tell him that it's okay to be sad. I actually wanted him to cry so I could give him "mummy hugs" and make it all better. But, absurdly, he was the one comforting me. If I cried he would put his arms round me but he didn't shed one single tear.

In reality, Adam wasn't coping very well at all and I think that food and exercise became his way of dealing with it. During the period between spring and summer 2011 I began to notice little things like quite a lot of his packed lunches were coming back from school. He'd taken just one bite out of his sandwich, that kind of thing. Later I found out that he was also throwing food away. But I really only noticed these warning signs with hindsight.

Around this time Adam weighed himself on a friend's weighing scales. The boy was a year older, yet Adam was heavier. It upset him a lot.

It didn't help that there was a heavy focus on healthy eating at school. At one point Adam was asked to keep a food diary for a week which, of course, made him look more closely at what he was consuming.

I am convinced that all these factors, although not "causes" of eating disorders (which are believed to be biologically-based mental illnesses and not a cultural phenomenon or lifestyle choice), definitely had an impact on Adam and probably helped to trigger his food restriction and exercise compulsion.

Anyway, there we were heading for MacDonald's on that day in early autumn 2011, immensely relieved that CAMHS felt that Adam was fine and that we were probably worrying over nothing.

I think we relaxed for a while, but pretty soon we could tell things weren't right. Adam seemed to be eating meals, but he'd play around with his food. He would never finish anything. It gradually got worse and worse. I remember saying to him something like: "I think you're eating too little again. Why is that?" And his answer chilled me to the bone: "Because I know how to." What a strange thing for a 10-year old boy to say. It didn't sound like Adam talking at all.

In the month following our CAMHS visit Adam dropped a further three kilos in weight. Unbeknown to us he was also revving up his exercise regime, especially after meals. He'd disappear up to his room and do hundreds of press-ups and leg lifts. Later he began to do star-jumps, too.

By now the alarm bells were ringing, so we called CAMHS, told them about everything, explained that he was losing weight and that his moods were getting worse. CAMHS called us back in. It was then that we discovered he'd lost the three kilos.

CAMHS admitted there was a problem, but still everyone seemed to be avoiding the "A" word. They gave him a meal plan which just made things worse. He couldn't stick to it. He told me the meal plan made him feel like a prisoner. He'd divide the food into tiny pieces, eat a bit and then leave the rest. He always had to leave some. It was awful. It was a really stressful time and things just got worse and worse.

The meal plan was more of a maintenance plan than a weight-gain plan. The thinking was that it would help Adam "get used to the idea" of having to eat properly. This seemed a reasonable suggestion at the time. After all, they were the experts and we thought they knew best. Why wouldn't we think this? But every time he gained a little weight he'd go and lose it again, sometimes losing even more. It became an awful cycle.

As parents we didn't know what we were supposed to do - or not do. I made it my mission to learn as much as I could about anorexia and eating disorders. I searched the internet for books and read as much as I could. I knew I needed to get a lot of food into my son, but it was proving to be much easier said than done.

By this stage we were "bargaining" with the illness saying things like: "If you eat this then we'll let you leave ten-per-cent of it." It just got ridiculous with Adam insisting that everything was weighed or measured meticulously.

It was really stressful. It was also incredibly distressing knowing that all of this was making Adam so very unhappy. I didn't want to make him unhappy so I thought that, by bargaining with the eating disorder, I'd eventually win him over. But it doesn't work like this. He just continued to lose weight.

Then, in January 2012 following more weight loss over a really terrible Christmas, CAMHS made the decision to admit Adam to the local adolescent eating disorders unit. He was only there full-time for a week or so. The trouble was, he'd gain some weight only to lose it all again, usually by exercising like mad in the bathroom. I was surprised that they allowed this to happen. But the emphasis was all about the patient "wanting to get better". Progress wouldn't be made until Adam got to the stage of "wanting to get better".

During Adam's inpatient stay I met another mother fighting this awful illness. She recommended the F.E.A.S.T. website and its Around The Dinner Table forum. Both of these became a lifeline to me during the darkest days. I could always go there and find help, advice and comfort from parents and carers who knew exactly how I felt.

When Adam was discharged he became a day patient. That was incredibly stressful for us, juggling our other children and school plus my husband's job and travelling to and from the hospital every day. They wanted me to do as many meals as possible with him. We'd usually do breakfast at home and then head for the hospital. The worst thing was that he wasn't getting any better.

I could have handled the stress if I'd noticed some improvement, but there just wasn't any. But at least I was a "full-time mum" so I could devote one-hundred-per-cent of my time to him. How parents and carers cope with full or even part-time jobs I have no idea.

I couldn't understand why the consultant didn't appear to be overly concerned about Adam's weight. It didn't seem to be a priority. I remember him saying something like: "There are some families where I'm concerned about the parents. There are some where I'm concerned about the child's weight. But with Adam I'm not concerned at all." Meanwhile I just couldn't make my son eat enough. I simply wasn't strong enough to do it. I was afraid of the eating disorder. I was afraid that if we pushed too hard then he wouldn't eat at all. And indeed that happened many times.

Diary Entry: Saturday 12th November 2011

Adam just asked me if I was sure I loved him. This was after lunch and we had to try and get him to finish a sausage. In the end he did, but then ran upstairs in a sulk and obviously very angry with me. I had tried to compromise with him as we were having a big lunch. I said he didn't have to have fruit and yogurt too. But he'd still have to have his snack later. I was trying to make him happier but it didn't work. I can live with him being angry with me. It's just seeing him so sad so much of the time that's so heartbreaking. It's been a very stressful week indeed. I can't think about anything else really. It's all consuming. He told me that he doesn't really want to do his exercises but feels awful if he doesn't. He does one set first thing; two sets after breakfast and lunch; another set after snack and another after tea. So he's increased his exercise by one set to compensate for the snack. (One set = 30 press-ups and 20 leg lifts.) He's been so upset today. Almost having a panic attack. He found it very hard to calm down. He's calm now though. I just need to stay strong through the difficult bits because he's mostly okay afterwards. I just want him to be happy. I wonder how long it'll take to get him better.

We had no effective deterrent or "Plan B" for food refusal. What we desperately wanted was to be able to say to Adam: "If you don't eat at home then you'll go into hospital where they will get you to eat, via a tube if necessary." CAMHS had their reasons why they didn't want to do this, but I never really understood why.

Things continued to yo-yo. Adam would gain a little and then he'd lose it again. Between that first appointment at CAMHS and when we parted company with CAMHS nine months later he'd lost more than seven kilos. And remember, he'd already lost weight before that. The illness certainly caused him to lose more than a quarter of his bodyweight in total, possibly as much as a third.

Absurdly, Adam felt sure he was gaining weight the whole time. He just saw the increases, not the decreases. Even a tiny 100g gain would upset him and he would redouble his exercise efforts to get it off. And every time he arrived at a new, lower weight that became his new maximum; the weight he was "happy" with and wouldn't go above. Even though the charts were showing a steep decline, he saw it all as weight gain. This just shows how much the illness can distort the patient's perceptions.

Diary Entry: Sunday 18th March 2012

It's Mothers' Day. Lovely card and present from Adam. The only present I want though, he can't give me. Colin is downstairs now struggling with porridge. Adam's mealtime behaviour is so bad at the moment. So sad. So resistant. If he's not lost weight again this week I'll be amazed.

So breakfast was torturous and then stopping him exercising. He was pacing and pacing so I physically held him and tried to get him to sit down - he fought and hit and kicked my shin. Between us we got him to sit down but he was kicking his legs. He can't sit still and paces when he stands. Eventually it was lunchtime and he sat down in great distress and immediately started picking bits off the sandwich. We told him to eat and then he just picked up the plate and threw the bits of sandwich at me and on the floor. I cleared up and I could have made another sandwich or just given him a build-up drink. We decided on the drink but he refused it - just pulled out the straw and threw it making a nice sticky mess. He was watching the girls play a computer game and totally ignoring us, so I said to Colin that he needed to go up on his bed. And that's where we are now. What a lovely Mothers' Day. Adam says he doesn't want to get better, doesn't want to put on weight and wants to die. We need to be as strong as we possibly can here. But how long will he refuse food?

Eventually it dawned on the clinicians that they weren't getting anywhere with Adam. They were worried about me, too. On a couple of occasions I'd run out of the room screaming because I just couldn't handle the fact that they didn't seem to be taking Adam's illness seriously. By now I was in a state of sheer panic. I had no idea where this was going. I could only see Adam getting worse and worse unless things changed drastically, and soon. From everything I'd read in books and on the F.E.A.S.T. website, I knew the only way to save Adam was to get his weight back to normal, and as quickly as possible. It was clear that this was not going to happen with CAMHS. I had been determined to re-feed Adam at home, but I felt like I was failing my son. Something had to change.

I'd heard of a private clinic that had been treating children and adolescents with eating disorders for 20 years or so. I knew of a couple of girls who had done very well there and I'd seen documentaries about it on TV. I thought: "Wow, we need to get Adam somewhere like this; I can't turn things around by myself at home." So I asked Adam's therapists if he could be referred there. Unfortunately they refused. They were also fairly scathing regarding the outcomes from "places like that". But they did suggest a second opinion from one of the big London NHS hospitals.

During this time I actually spoke to the private clinic who offered Adam a place. The team at the London hospital were really good, too, when we saw them - they agreed that getting weight on Adam was an absolute priority and that inpatient care was needed as it looked unlikely that we could turn things round at home. However, they didn't have any beds available. So we made the decision to go private.

The regime at the private clinic was very strict, the focus being on weight gain. They took Adam in, stopped all his exercise and monitored him closely to make sure he wasn't exercising in secret. Adam also had to eat. He was allowed privileges whenever he was on track for his target weight. But to get those privileges he also had to finish his meals within a certain time and not exercise. Privileges were things like being allowed to go on walks or trips, or just to go on the swings in the garden. I remember Adam being so happy the first time he was allowed on the swings! Parents are initially excluded from the treatment and we were only permitted to visit once a week. However I could speak to him over the phone every night. It sounds draconian, but it worked. Also, being separated from us meant that there were none of the bad habits you develop as a parent battling with your child's eating disorder at home, for example the bargaining and that kind of thing.

The programme at this particular private clinic is very structured. To start with, parents are not involved at all with meals or eating. This is actually excellent, and such a relief, as it takes all that stress and guilt away. As the child gains weight and meets the other requirements, such as finishing meals on time and not exercising, then parents are gradually brought back in to handle meals. It starts with picnics building up to restaurant meals and eventually weekends at home. All these tasks must be passed before moving on to the next one, and all have to be completed before the child is discharged. It works amazingly well. Well it did for Adam at any rate after a rather shaky start (because he found it so hard to stop exercising).

But despite the shaky start I could see him getting better every week. It was amazing. He was in there for 14 weeks altogether. We were so very, very fortunate that Colin's private medical insurance paid for it all and continued to fund on-going outpatient therapy afterwards.

The aftercare was fantastic. They have something called Weekend Return. The idea is that you have to stick to their rules whilst at home and can call them if you have any problems. The patient's weight is monitored and if they're losing again, then they're admitted for a weekend. As long as you send in the patient's weight every week, and take the hospital's advice if you have problems, then this facility is available for as long as you need it. While Adam was there, a boy who had been discharged many months earlier came back in on Weekend Return. I think this sent a powerful message to Adam. Thankfully Adam never had to go back.

Now, five or six months on from being discharged, Adam is doing really well. He eats everything we want him to eat. He still has issues, for instance he is almost phobic of eating in front of anyone other than his family. He will only eat what we tell him to and he never has anything "extra". And if I don't pay him one-hundred-per-cent attention at mealtimes, he'll stop eating. Having said this, we are in a really good place now. I can definitely see little green shoots and less rigidity in his behaviour. Things are starting to shift and Adam is now a healthy weight, so our story has a happy ending.

As for me, well, I know what I'm doing now. I'm with him for almost every meal he has. The exercise addiction took a while to solve at the private clinic. Adam kept getting penalised for exercising in the night or jiggling around. It was really hard for him. Eventually he was allowed an hour's exercise each day and he's happy with these parameters because it helps him keep it in line.

The exercise addiction was horrendous. He hated exercising but felt compelled to do it. He couldn't go to school if he hadn't done all his sit-ups and crunches. At one point I remember him being so tired, thin and ill that he could barely do the exercises. But he couldn't be "happy" unless he'd done them, so he ploughed ahead.

One thing that helped me enormously was the F.E.A.S.T. website and the Around The Dinner Table forum. Through this I found dozens of parents who'd been through similar experiences, including parents of boys with eating disorders, and I've made a lot of lasting friends through this forum. Thinking about it, we F.E.A.S.Ties, as we call ourselves these days, are quite a force to be reckoned with when it comes to promoting evidence-based treatment of eating disorders. I've learned an incredible amount from the other parents there. I really do credit them, along with the private clinic, for helping me to save my precious son's life.

Natalie's story

"The A&E nurse said: 'I'll go and get you a glass of squash; it won't be too much.' And there I was trying to explain that my daughter wouldn't even drink water, let alone squash."

It's funny how anorexia isolates its victims and transforms them physically and mentally into people we don't recognise. No, it's not funny at all; it's heart-breaking, especially when it's your own child.

If you'd seen Jessica before she became ill, you would have seen someone who was fun-loving, outgoing and who loved being with her friends. She had a wicked sense of humour; in fact she had a really evil sense of humour! She was a great one for mucking in and joining in with anything that was going on with the family. She was also very sporty. In fact she'd been sporty from a young age. But then, very gradually and almost without me noticing, things began to change.

Around the age of 14 she began to want to be more independent and do less with the family. Initially we thought: "Oh, it's just typical teens." But then in the November, shortly before she turned 15, I discovered that she'd begun to self-harm. She was cutting her thighs, arms and tummy and, on one occasion, I was horrified to see that she had carved the words F-A-T into her tummy and thighs. I immediately challenged her about it and she said she was having problems with some of the girls at school; that they were pushing her away, that kind of thing. She also had a friend who'd become very depressed and Jessica said she felt like a failure because she couldn't do anything to help this friend. Suddenly it was as if everything was happening at once. But I didn't suspect an emerging eating disorder because, at the time, she was eating normally.

Shortly after turning 15, Jessica began to exercise more intensively, running and cycling after school in addition to her usual swimming (as a club swimmer she was already training for 90 minutes four times a week). She claimed the extra exercise was to help with the swimming; she was worried that she wasn't keeping up with the other girls in her age group. Initially we didn't think anything of it. When I was Jessica's age I used to very sporty and she appeared to be taking after me.

It wasn't until she began to cut back on what she was eating that the alarm bells really began to ring. Over the next three months, Jessica began to cut out puddings. She'd ask for smaller helpings of main meals and refuse foods that were high in fat. We also discovered she'd been giving away her packed lunch for a few months. Then she stopped eating breakfast. By now she was living on just one tiny meal a day.

Meanwhile her moods were getting worse and would swing from one extreme to the other. One moment she would be happily joining in with whatever the family was doing and the next she'd be slamming doors and refusing to talk, accusing us of "not caring" and "not loving" her, that we "didn't know what it was like" and to leave her alone. I was concerned, especially with the self-harm that was going on, but she was seeing a counsellor for this at school. The school explained that a number of girls in her year group had been self-harming. The counsellor said that if she felt more help was needed then she would get in touch with us. So we thought all right, fine, it's under control.

But in the New Year things began to get worse, almost by the week. Suddenly everything began to happen so very quickly. The weight began to drop off her, quite dramatically. She was having trouble sleeping, her moods were getting worse and she was self-harming more than ever.

Curiously, although Jessica was eating very little, she became increasingly interested in cooking. I've always been a keen cook and always have lots of recipes and magazines around the house. Jessica would grab the magazines, rip out the recipe pages and spirit them away to a box up in her room. I had no idea until I discovered the box one day. She began cooking, mainly sweet things: cakes, biscuits, scones and things like that. But she never ate any of it.

I became terrified. I felt isolated. I was also angry with myself for not spotting it sooner. By now the penny had dropped. Jessica was developing an eating disorder. The symptoms were as clear as day. I know because I used to have anorexia as a teenager although I guess I was what you might call a "failed anorexic" in that I loved food too much. In the end I became bulimic. The eating disorder was still a problem after I married and had the kids, but I was always careful to hide it well. No-one ever knew what was going on. Eventually I got help and am now in remission. But, as it became more and more clear that Jessica was developing an eating disorder, I felt incredibly guilty. Had I, in some way, "passed it on" to my beautiful, intelligent daughter? Had I not been as careful in hiding the bulimia as I thought I had?

As Jessica deteriorated, I became desperate for help. I knew of the eating disorders charity Beat, but felt that nowhere covered our unique family scenario: me with multiple health issues, in and out of hospital up to ten times a year, plus my eating disorder history. I felt incredibly alone, especially as friends just responded with comments like: "Don't worry; she'll grow out of it." I'm sure they thought I was over-reacting, but I knew deep down that things were seriously wrong.

Jessica lost weight rapidly and within six months went from eating well to having just a tiny meal in the evening. Meanwhile she'd exercise whenever she could, and kept herself so isolated and withdrawn that it was hard to have a conversation with her. I knew we had to get help.

Initially I met with our GP alone. I told her of my concerns about the weight loss, low moods, self-harm and isolation. She listened and agreed that there could be an issue. Jessica then joined us in the surgery to be weighed and measured. Next, the GP spoke to Jessica alone. Unfortunately Jessica wasn't very communicative so the doctor didn't find out much.

I felt that, although the GP had listened to me, she hadn't really taken on board how worried I was. She did say that it "could" be the start of anorexia. On the other hand it might be "just a phase" due to stresses at school. Also, because Jessica's periods surprisingly hadn't stopped by this point, I was told that - although she was underweight - it wasn't serious. This still haunts our family to this day. To Jessica, having periods means she isn't ill and certainly not anorexic.

Anyway, the GP told us to come back in a month. Then three weeks later my own health problems deteriorated and I was admitted to hospital. When Jessica visited me a few days later her weight loss was so obvious that my husband made an urgent appointment with a different GP for the following day. This GP weighed her and noted that she'd lost weight since her last visit. The doctor had a long chat with my husband and then rang CAMHS. We were given an appointment for a week's time - an assessment to decide what kind of treatment would be most appropriate - and told that if we were at all concerned, we must take Jessica to A&E.

Following the CAMHS assessment Jessica was urgently referred to a large adolescent eating disorders clinic for a further assessment. Thankfully Jessica was given an appointment for the end of that week. Even then we had to take Jessica to A&E as she hadn't eaten or drunk anything for five days.

The staff at A&E were pretty ineffective, treating Jessica like a small child and saying inappropriate things. For example on learning that Jessica was refusing to eat or drink, the nurse said: "I'll go and get you a glass of squash; it won't be too much." And there I was trying to explain that my daughter wouldn't even drink water, let alone squash.

I got the impression that they had no knowledge of eating

disorders whatsoever. The duty psychiatrist wasn't much better. He said: "Well, if you'll eat something in front of me then you can go home."

I said: "Why on earth would she eat anything in front of you? She won't eat anything in front of anyone, not her parents, not her sisters, not even her grandparents." But it was all a bit like: "Well you've got the appointment coming up at the eating disorders clinic, so why did you bring her here?" And I responded with: "Well, if *your* child hadn't eaten or drunk anything for five whole days wouldn't *you* seek emergency help?" By now I was absolutely seething. But we were sent back home.

Anyhow, the day of the appointment at the eating disorders clinic arrived. Jessica was assessed and we were told that she needed urgent treatment. A further appointment was made for four days' time. Before she left the centre, Jessica was given a build-up drink, the first of many battles with those little calorie-laden drinks!

Looking back, although - as a former sufferer of an eating disorder - I knew what to look out for, I'm baffled at the way I didn't recognise the early signs in Jessica until her anorexia was much more advanced. Another thing that was new to me, despite my own battles with eating disorders, was the impact that these illnesses have on the family, especially when it's your own child that's suffering. Until Jessica fell ill, I had no idea how isolating having a child with mental health problems could be. In the early days friends and family were supportive, but this support soon began to fade away.

One of the other things that shocked me was just how long a simple trip to the supermarket could take with Jessica in tow. It could take three times as long as going on my own. Yet I had to take her with me; by now she wasn't in a fit state to be left at home alone and her dad was working shifts.

She'd pick up and examine the nutritional labelling of anything that she might even vaguely consider eating. She'd get out her phone, stand in the middle of the supermarket and tap away on it trying to work out how many calories and fat units there were in a portion. If I put things into the trolley that she didn't want to eat, she'd put them back onto the shelf. I'd get desperate, scouring the supermarket trying to find something she would eat. Meanwhile I'd watch other people pushing their trolleys around the supermarket shopping as normal. It made me feel angry and frustrated.

I knew that eating disorders were manipulative but I never really understood how much damage they caused to the family. There I was, living under the same roof as my daughter, yet it was as if I no longer recognised her. I'd often go to bed wondering if she'd still be alive the next morning. Our lives were put on hold and the family ended up splitting up - and all because of this horrible illness.

Treatment at the eating disorders clinic was intensive and included a number of admissions as an inpatient, all of which were incredibly traumatic for the whole family. I can't even begin to describe what it's like to see your beloved, beautiful daughter so very, very thin, being fed through a tube, and so distressed that she attempted to take her own life on more than one occasion.

Yet, to our delight and surprise, in the summer she sat her GCSE examinations and achieved five passes, despite no formal schooling in over a year.

In the September, Jessica was allowed out of the unit on day release to ease herself back into school. But she just couldn't do it. Her self-esteem and confidence had completely disappeared. The next few months were a real struggle. Then, in the following March, she was discharged home on condition that she underwent weekly DBT sessions (Dialectical Behaviour Therapy) and medical monitoring. Her diet was still very restrictive, her weight was still very low and, as a result of the anorexia, her moods and emotions were haywire.

Jessica is still a "work in progress". I find it so frustrating that, two years down the line, we still have so far to go. She's still eating a limited number of calories and foodstuffs, and as far as I'm aware her weight hasn't gone up; indeed it looks as if it's going down. She hasn't let us weigh her for about six weeks now.

I'm sorry that I can't be more positive at this stage. But what I can say is that I now know more about eating disorders and their treatment than I ever did before, despite my own history of anorexia and bulimia. And we have a fantastic team of clinicians behind us. Basically we'll do whatever it takes to ensure our daughter gets well, and stays well; it's what families do. It's hard work, but we'll do it.

MY TIPS:

Get support for yourself. One of the many things I wish I'd done sooner is to join the ATDT forum. The support I have found there is truly amazing. (See list of resources at the end of the book.)

Use all the professional help you can get your hands on. And please don't be afraid to ask for a second opinion if you feel uncomfortable at any time. Never forget, it's your child's life that's at stake.

Separate your child from their illness. Remember that behind the illness your daughter or son is still there and they are scared and frightened, too. Always allow them time to talk, even if it's at 4am. Always tell them you love them but hate the illness.

Look after yourself. You need to be fit and well, in body and spirit, to be able to help your child. Also, accept all help in whatever form it comes. Don't forget about yourself and the rest of the family. Yes, your sick child needs you but so does the rest of the family. Ask others to help out to allow this to happen.

Trust your instinct. If you have any concerns go to your GP as soon as possible and keep pestering them until they take you seriously. Early on I was told I was over-reacting. I began to wonder if I was. And that slowed down the diagnosis at a critical time.

Trust others' instincts. If anyone else voices concerns about your child take them seriously. Often when you live with an eating disorder day to day you don't see things until it's too late.

Educate friends and family and enlist their support.

Distraction works. Try to distract your child from what they are eating and also after meals with banter, TV, games - anything.

Keep your child safe. Ensure your child's room is as safe as possible - I had to remove all sharp objects, etc.

Be aware of "false summits". I wish I'd known how deceiving the illness can be with its peaks and troughs. There have been so many times I thought I was seeing the light at the end of the tunnel when - ping! - we'd find ourselves back at Square One.

Get as much support as possible from the school and other activities your child is involved in. If possible try and encourage your child not to cut themselves off from the world.

Don't blame yourself - I know how hard this is but your child's eating disorder is not your fault.

Eva's story

"We parents know we have to get our children to eat. We know what they need to eat and how much of it they need to eat. The problem is, *how* do we get them to eat?"

When my daughter, Katie, was discharged from inpatient treatment for her anorexia, I was expected to continue feeding her at home, just as she'd been fed at the hospital: three meals and three snacks a day. Yet I had no idea how to help her to eat if she wasn't at least a little bit willing. Despite asking over and over again how I should feed my child, the response always seemed to be a kind of cheerful and confident: "You're the parents; you're perfectly capable. Don't worry, you'll find a way!"

I only wish it had been that simple!

Eventually our eating disorders service agreed to send some FBT (Family-Based Treatment) specialists round to our house. They observed a couple of meals and gave us practical advice on how to feed Katie. It made all the difference. So much so that I believe that if they'd done it 12 months earlier we might have saved my daughter a year of hospital treatment. And one year is a big chunk out of a young person's life.

Katie's anorexia first began to emerge in the spring of 2009 when she was 10 years old. Up to then she'd been a perfectly normal girl brought up in a happy and stable environment. Then in March 2009 a minor bullying incident set her off dieting. She'd fallen out with some friends and they'd chanted to her that she was fat. So she'd decided she needed to get thin, even though she'd never been fat in the first place.

Looking back, we often wonder if there were other clues, too. For some time, every six months or so, she'd been asking us if she looked fat. Then she developed this strange fixation with death and would worry about us dying in a car crash whenever we went out. Were these clues? Certainly the experts couldn't say to us that, oh yes, those were clear signs.

I knew about the bullying because Katie had told me about it. But what she didn't tell me was that she'd begun to restrict her food. By May 2009 the "Am I fat?" questions had become much more frequent. She'd also begun to refuse some snacks saying that she didn't "need them". And if we went out to a café, for instance, she'd take an awful long time to make a decision and then beat herself up about it afterwards. She'd say things like: "Am I fat? I shouldn't have eaten that. I'm really stuffed."

So, by this time, I was aware that she was trying to diet. But I also knew that most of the girls in her group were flirting with diets; it was all the rage, even for girls as young as 10. I just assumed her obsession with food and body shape would pass as soon as I'd managed to steer her away from dieting.

By the middle of July I was beginning to panic, concerned that we didn't have much time to play with. We seemed to be forever having conversations about food and being fat. Katie would ask endless questions like: "Have I eaten too much? How do you know I haven't eaten too much?" In fact during that two month period between May and July my thinking had undergone a massive shift from "I'm worried about Katie dieting on the sly" to "This is serious. I'm really worried and we need to get this fixed urgently".

By this stage I'd read a couple of books which made me pretty sure she had anorexia. But I was worried about telling Katie. I was concerned that "labelling" her with anorexia might make things worse. This is what made us delay taking her to the GP even though I was getting extremely worried. I was still hoping that I could fix it at home without the need for any medical intervention.

Over the next few days I became conscious that we were on a horrible downward spiral. So my husband and I made a deal with Katie. We agreed that she needn't put on any weight as long as she ate whatever we gave her, which would be exactly the right amount for her to remain static. What she mustn't do was to lose any more weight.

With hindsight I know this was a crazy deal that could never have worked. And of course it didn't. Katie would complain that she felt so full she felt sick, so she couldn't possibly eat all that food. So she continued to lose weight even though, in theory, she'd agreed on the deal.

By this stage she'd become a total zombie. She was depressed. We couldn't engage her in any kind of distraction or hobby which wasn't a sport. She just sat or stood in her room staring into space. At least that's what we thought. The truth is that when we weren't watching she was driven to exercise. Handstands were her favourite.

Everything was happening at such a terrifying pace that, by the end of July, I was getting frantic. I knew we needed outside help urgently so, initially, I went to see our GP on my own. I was still worried that whatever the GP said would somehow put a spanner in the works if my daughter was "labelled" as having anorexia.

I described the endless questions about weight and how she'd ask things like: "How do you know you're not giving me too much food?" I explained how she'd say: "I've eaten too much!" and "I look fat!" I told her about the way Katie's skin was dry, her eyes were hollow, her lips were thin and her hands were freezing cold; in fact the way she was constantly complaining of being cold even though it was midsummer. I told the GP that Katie looked like a zombie, was utterly depressed and couldn't engage with anything. I described how her only happy moments recently were linked to exercise.

The GP said that, yes, it really did sound as if she had anorexia and that we had to take this very seriously. She asked me to bring Katie in to be weighed and measured; meanwhile she would prepare a referral so that we didn't waste any time.

Looking back, I'm really glad I'd read all those books on eating disorders because it enabled me to go along to the GP and present her with a clear list of symptoms. We were also fortunate to have a GP who could recognise anorexia and knew that intervention was urgently required. My advice to other parents would be to take a list of symptoms along with you to the GP. Also, bear in mind that even though your child may not look like a skeleton, it doesn't mean they don't have anorexia. Katie wasn't skeletal by this time. She was thin, yes, but not overly so.

So a few days later I took Katie to see the GP.

Katie had prepared a list of questions like: "How do I know I'm not too fat?" But the GP simply said: "I'm going to weigh and measure you, check that you're safe and then I will refer you to a specialist. Are you OK with that?"

We waited for the referral to come through, but heard nothing. So for several days I was making frantic phone calls, only to find that we'd been referred to an obsolete service instead of CAMHS. This probably added a week's delay to the proceedings.

A week might not sound too serious. But because of the way things were spiralling out of control, a week's delay was horrendous. By now Katie's fluid intake was minimal; she'd just about drink a cup of milk a day if we were lucky and very little water. Sometimes I'd manage to get a stew or some soup into her but by mid-August it was just the milk, nothing else. In fact she was so dehydrated by this point that, when she was called in for a blood test, they couldn't find a vein to draw blood from.

By this stage Katie had become very obsessive, too. She'd become obsessed about germs, for example. If I touched a piece of food she was about to eat she'd be horrified. By September, taking a shower required all her courage, as her undernourished brain told her that water might make her fat. This kind of freakish obsessive behaviour evaporated as soon as she began to eat properly again and gain weight.

Desperate to get her into "the system", I called CAMHS who said they'd received the referral. Katie had been assessed as a priority and would be seen as soon as possible, either this week or next. Otherwise, according to them, it would have been a two-year wait!

Thankfully the first CAMHS appointment came through a few days later.

It was a Wednesday. They told us that if, by Friday, Katie hadn't eaten and drunk enough she would be admitted to hospital. On that day I managed to get three quarters of a cup of water into her by mid-afternoon but that was the best I could do. No food. So we were absolutely desperate. But the threat of hospital prompted her to eat a bit. She'd been told she had to have three meals and three snacks a day. It was all very clear.

Katie did eat - just enough to muddle through. But it really was muddling through.

After that first appointment we had a meeting at least once a week and the CAMHS nurse coordinator was happy for us to phone any time. She was great, actually. We also had a CAMHS psychiatrist and a dietician, so at this stage we really felt that we had a good support team in place. Hopefully, we thought to ourselves optimistically, we'll begin to see some positive changes very soon.

At the end of August CAMHS threatened hospital again. So, at home, we worked really hard to feed her. Slowly but surely Katie was beginning to eat more. It was becoming a bit less desperate. But just as we thought things were starting to move in the right direction, she came down with a tummy bug. She didn't eat for a couple of days. I don't know if this set off the spiral again - and we'll never know if we could have fixed things at home if it hadn't been for the tummy bug - but it really came at a terrible time.

She got worse and began to cut down even more on her food. So we were back in a real emergency situation. Our relationship with her was often confrontational because we were trying so hard to get her to eat but we just didn't have the skills to do it. I'd go online and Google things like: "How do I feed my child?" I knew I had to feed her; that was really obvious. But what I didn't know was *how*. My husband and I would swing from one extreme to another, from: "We've got to insist she eats what we give her" to "No, this is creating so many fights. She's getting more entrenched. We've got to be much more soft and gentle with her. As long as she eats enough to be safe then let's leave it at that." In our ignorance, we thought that psychological interventions would be the key to getting our daughter to eat.

Very quickly we got to the stage where we realised that the psychiatric inpatient unit was going to save her life. We'd heard from other people that it was a nice ward; it was very homely and small, just four to six children in it at any one time. It wasn't *One flew over the cuckoo's nest* by any stretch of the imagination. The CAMHS nurse coordinated the admission beautifully.

We had a pre-admission visit in the middle of September. I was so reassured at how friendly the staff were and how the psychiatrist and all the other people in charge were so non-blaming. Even though it wasn't a specialist eating disorders unit - it was a general under 12s mental health unit - they had plenty of experience with anorexic children. They knew that the illness wasn't my daughter's fault, that she was very scared and that she needed a lot of support. So that really put my mind at rest. I didn't want her to be locked away in a punitive, scary environment.

Following the visit Katie was desperate to go into the unit and did everything she could to accelerate her admission. She stopped eating and more or less stopped drinking. I took her to A&E on one occasion to get her checked out, but mainly so I could get her to drink in front of a doctor. I think she just wanted to get out of the house and into the hospital. By this stage the anorexia was raging.

She was admitted at the end of September and remained in the unit for nearly a year.

Right from the start we were involved in her care. The hospital asked us to visit every day. Even if Katie tried to send us away or didn't want to talk to us, we still needed to be there. So that's what we did. Actually it was really easy compared to the nightmare we'd been living over the last few months and the unit was only 20 minutes' drive away.

The aim was that Katie would gradually get what they call "home passes" and that she would steadily spend more and more time at home. The problem was that she was terrified of coming home. She felt safe in the unit. The nurses were kind and they made eating easy. She was having fun; she was able to distract herself from her illness. She played with the other kids, she felt secure and she ate everything they put in front of her. We couldn't believe it. We were waiting for the tide to turn and for her to refuse food, but she never did.

Basically, Katie was given no option but to eat. The staff just seemed to have a knack of getting her to eat and it was something my husband and I were desperate to learn how to do at home. The nurses were also aware of all the tricks that anorexia patients can play to pull the wood over the clinicians' eyes. Once, when they caught her exercising in the shower, they insisted that for a few weeks she'd have to shower with the door open. The illness was never permitted to get the upper hand.

One downside was that the hospital fed her only the foods that she agreed to have on her eating plan. As a result she became pretty regimented in her eating. There were no fear foods on the plan, just the few odd foods she felt comfortable with. She maintained a safe weight but her mind set remained anorexic.

As time went on she was able to spend several days at a time at home. She was also attending school for three days a week. School representatives came to the case conferences held by the hospital, and so did the outpatient team and the GP. In this way, when Katie was discharged from the ward at the end of August 2010, the handover was very smooth.

The outpatient team now included CAMHS and an eating disorders unit using Family-Based Treatment (FBT). The eating disorders unit was supported via Skype by a team led by FBT expert Dr Daniel Le Grange in the US.

Katie was an outpatient for nearly a year. By the time she was discharged she was really well. She wasn't totally "cured"; she still needed us to tell her what to eat and she still watched how much she was eating. But by then we knew what we were doing and trusted that time would do the rest, so we were happy with the discharge.

In summary, Katie benefited from prompt diagnosis and life-saving care in the psychiatric ward. After a period of stagnation there, she made rapid progress back home with Family-Based Treatment. Looking back, the main thing that delayed Katie's recovery was the lack of coaching on how we, as parents, should go about feeding our child at home. It was only because I kept pleading that the FBT therapists agreed to observe us in our home and give us practical advice. It made all the difference. It meant that we were then able, at last, to systematically expose Katie to the foods she feared, and she improved very quickly. I believe that if we'd had this coaching 12 months earlier we might have saved the NHS a year of costly hospitalisation, not to mention accelerating Katie's recovery.

I also wish our clinicians had been able to teach us how to rebuild a close and trusting relationship with Katie, because it took me a long time to find other sources of help. The emotional aspects, and the "how to" around feeding, were so instrumental to Katie's recovery that - once she was well - I decided to write a book and share with other parents all the tools that made such a difference.

Another thing I wish I'd done earlier was to sign up to the Around The Dinner Table forum which supports parents of young people with eating disorders. I'd actually discovered the forum and its "parent" website F.E.A.S.T. quite early on in Katie's illness, but at the time I was wary of forums. It was only when I began to write my book that I clicked back onto the forum, had a look around and thought: "Wow! This is really good!" I really wish I'd paid more attention to it during those early days because I would have had a stack of answers.

Obviously I would have had the moral support of the forum, too, and would have discovered that my daughter wasn't at all unusual.

Because she'd been in hospital for so long we were convinced that her case was particularly severe, but on the forum I found lots of families that had been through similar experiences.

So, apart from a few regrets, our story is one of care ranging from competent to excellent, with a very happy ending.

Now, aged 14, Katie shows no signs of anorexia and although I will probably remain discretely vigilant for a while, everything's back to normal and life is good.

Martha's story

"As a parent, I have not felt listened to during the whole of my daughter's illness. We may not be 'experts' but we still know our children best. And eating disorders appear to be one area of medicine where parental opinions are regularly ignored."

I remember looking at Francesca, just as she'd begun to go through puberty. She was beginning to fill out a bit. She'd developed a waist, a bust and curves, and I remember thinking: "I wonder if she'll think she's fat." She wasn't fat, of course. She was quite small-framed and she'd always been a picky eater. But it was just a fleeting thought and I thought no more of it.

Looking back, though, she'd begun to "eat healthily" at the beginning of secondary school. I think it was something to do with all the talk about healthy eating that was going on at the time. She'd also seen a film about battery chickens and had decided to go vegetarian. But, really, she was absolutely normal. She had bags of energy and she'd go through the normal growth spurts.

It wasn't until she was around the age of 15 that I began to notice she was getting depressed. The eating disorder probably crept in at this time, too, but I was primarily concerned with the depression. The eating side of things didn't really register. I remember her coming down with a virus and she lost her appetite for a while. Then she just stopped eating breakfast and that's when I started to think: "Something isn't right here."

One day I remember her just sitting and crying, saying: "I'm just

111

so useless at everything, I can't do anything." It was so unlike her because she'd always been so positive. This really caused me concern because I remembered back to when I'd been her age and had been very depressed. So already I was thinking: "Things aren't quite right." I mean, she was eating; she just wasn't eating as much as she should be. Other people began to notice how thin she was getting. I think I didn't notice so much because I was with her all the time. Then I suddenly began to panic that an eating disorder was setting in. I didn't know anything about anorexia but I just had a strong hunch that something was going wrong.

I took her to the doctor who weighed her and said her BMI was a bit low. He sent her to see a community dietician where Francesca announced: "Oh, 500 calories a day is enough for my needs!" 500 calories? You wouldn't feed a small child on that, let alone a 15-year old growing girl.

By now I knew that things were badly wrong so I took her back to the GP. Francesca would complain that she just couldn't eat and that she felt "full" all the time. The GP wondered whether there was a physical cause. But by this time I was really panicking. I felt that we couldn't risk hanging around, waiting for appointments for a physical examination. I was getting really worried.

Fortunately there was a psychiatric nurse at the school where I worked. I told her that Francesca was losing weight fast. She suggested I went back to the GP who agreed to refer Francesca to CAMHS. I was still thinking that depression lay at the root of all this. I actually thought that the reason she'd stopped eating was a very slow suicide, as a result of being depressed. This is what I thought was going on in her head because she was so "not right".

Anyway, the psychiatric nurse colleague helped to fast-track us through the system. But when our CAMHS appointment came up, Francesca refused to go. I told her she had to go. I was in tears. It was awful. I remember us getting as far as the hospital car park, then Francesca just sitting there, refusing to get out of the car. In the end I shouted: "You're getting out of that car and going to that appointment even if I have to drag you along!" I was desperate.

Meanwhile she'd virtually stopped eating apart from little scraps. Oh, and she was drinking a lot of water. The weight was just falling off her. When I eventually got her into CAMHS we found ourselves in a room with a nurse, and a psychiatrist who took Francesca off for a chat. On her return, she said that, yes, Francesca was suffering from anorexia and that she had to get onto an eating regime of three meals and three snacks a day. The psychiatrist explained that Francesca would have a voice in her head "telling her not to eat". She said that if Francesca *couldn't* eat, then she would be admitted as an inpatient.

Okay, I thought to myself, I'm going to get her to eat. And for the first week I actually managed to do it and she held her weight. In fact she held it for a couple of weeks. I asked the psychiatrist what I should do next. How much should I increase her intake by? The psychiatrist simply said: "I don't know." And so I had no direction. I didn't know how to move things forward. As a result I simply couldn't get any weight onto her at home. Francesca, well, she'd already come to terms with the fact that she'd have to go into hospital and within a month she was admitted to a private eating disorders unit where her care was funded by the NHS. Things had moved so very fast between January and the end of May that I could hardly catch my breath.

Francesca put on weight in the unit. In fact they pushed her to quite a high weight, far higher than her pre-eating disorder weight. So I felt a bit uneasy and I know that Francesca found this very difficult to handle.

I often wonder whether it was this that was responsible for her relapse. I know it's all well and good looking back and saying we should have done this, that and the other, but the main frustration for me was that I wasn't listened to as a parent. Also, I wanted her to be given *Diazepam* to calm her down a bit and help her anxiety around eating, but instead they sectioned her under the Mental Health Act for a month and then forcibly tube-fed her. I don't have a problem with that but I wish they'd tried medication first. I just believe it would have made things a little easier and would have helped Francesca to manage her anxiety. I felt they weren't listening to me on two counts: medication and weight target. When she came out of hospital the psychiatrist reluctantly prescribed *Fluoxetine* and she was really quite well on it for a few months.

Unfortunately when Francesca came out of the unit she came down with a bad tummy bug which, of course, resulted in lost weight. Unfortunately this set off the restricting cycle again. At this time I was frantically scouring the internet to find anything I could about eating disorders. Much of what I was reading claimed there was a psychological explanation for anorexia. Indeed our psychiatrist had said: "This is all about the death of her father." (My husband had passed away when Francesca was five, more than ten years before.)

Now, that didn't make sense to me. I'd done so much work with Francesca over the years about her dad's death. Instinct told me that the eating disorder wasn't psychological. If it had been, I am sure I could have got through to her more easily. As it was, when I saw the resistance to eating and everything else… the facial expressions, the tone of her voice, everything… it struck me that this had to be something that was *physically* wrong with the brain; it wasn't just psychological.

That was when I came across the F.E.A.S.T. website and suddenly my instincts began to make sense. I also got hold of Lock and Le Grange's book *Help Your Teenager Beat an Eating Disorder* which talks about how you can get into a cycle of hospitalisation and that each hospitalisation can get longer. I then understood that Francesca had to learn to eat outside of the hospital setting. I had to de-institutionalise her and I needed to feed her at home.

The second time she was in hospital I made a point of telling them that, once she'd arrived at a "safe weight", I'd be taking her home and continuing to re-feed her there, outside the institutionalised routine of a hospital setting. The staff didn't like this, but I did it because I felt it was the right thing to do. Together she and I worked at it. And we made good progress.

We went on holiday and I was delighted to see she'd put on weight by the time we got back. The next two or three months were very positive, too. She started at a new school and continued to put on weight. But then, unfortunately, we went on another holiday and she lost weight again.

We went back to CAMHS on our return, but I was alarmed at the way it was interpreted, as if losing this weight had been "her choice" or "her fault". They wouldn't listen to me when I said we'd been working really well together and that we'd established a successful regime between the two of us. Yes, she'd lost weight on holiday, but I knew that together, with CAMHS' backing, we could get it back on and begin to move forward again.

But they weren't listening to me. And because I didn't get the backing I so needed from them, the successful regime collapsed. It's just one example of why everyone - parents and clinicians - need to be on the same page, working together as a tight-knit team against the eating disorder. I remember saying in exasperation: "Will you not tell her to eat?" The psychiatrist's response was: "Oh no, we just don't do that. Francesca has to take responsibility for her own health."

After that, I simply couldn't get things back on track and we stagnated for the best part of a year. I then transferred her care to the GP who was happy to take her on with the caveat that if she continued to lose weight then she was to go back to CAMHS. So the two of us just kept chugging along, really.

She did get transferred to Adult Services once she reached the age of 18. She saw a dietician there and a very nice psychiatrist. But, after a couple of months, the dietician told Francesca: "You're not working with me so there's no point in you coming along." So she felt abandoned and we continued to muddle through, just the two of us.

These days, Francesca's weight is still low, but she understands that she needs to have three meals and three snacks a day. The good news is that she can be flexible around meal times, she can eat on her own and she eats out with friends regularly. She is now at university and is under the local eating disorders service. The nurse is good but, again, the dietician gave up on her after a while. I worry that they're just not engaging with her; they're busy trying to address the rigidity and behaviours whereas, in my mind, these will fade away if they get the weight back onto her and the brain is given time to heal. But, because her weight is still low and she's finding it very hard to stick to their particular regime, she's being treated like a bit of a naughty girl and she hates that. She also refuses to attend group lunches where the centre prepares the food which is part of a new "programme" they introduced recently. She would far rather make her own meal arrangements, however she is not at a stage where she is able to do this yet.

The good thing is that we both like the new psychiatrist who is not at all judgmental. She has shown that she is open to my requests and that she will be willing to support us however we want to move things forward. Basically if Francesca wants to go back into hospital for a short period the psychiatrist will support this. She has also said that she is willing to prescribe *Diazepam* if Francesca wants to try it.

So, in spite of everything, Francesca is living a pretty normal life, enjoying her studies and managing to work. She's doing her essays, looking forward to her next nursing placement and is riding both at home and at university, which she loves. And we appear finally to have found a clinician who she can relate to. Up to now, the one clinician who she did get on with, and she got on with her very well, was the psychotherapist at the hospital, but once she'd been discharged she wasn't permitted to continue the relationship. To me this seemed absurd.

With this new psychiatrist, I finally feel that we can start moving things forward again - but it has been a long time coming. I have not felt listened to as a parent during the whole of this illness - and to me that is ridiculous. We may not be "experts" but we parents still know our children best. And eating disorders appear to be one area of medicine where parental opinions are regularly ignored.

Tanya's story

"I remember going out to a restaurant and Lauren ordering a huge meal and a massive pudding with ice cream. It really was amazing, because she ate everything she was served up!"

Remember when there was that drive about healthy eating? When getting your "five a day" was drilled into us all via the media? I think that's when it all started for my eldest daughter, Lauren. She'd be about 13 back then and I distinctly remember her exclaiming with delight that: "Look, mummy, I've had my five a day!" And then it would be: "Look, mummy, I've had *ten* of my five a day!" She was very concerned about having enough fruit and vegetables. Meanwhile she was exercising like mad. She'd do things like insist on walking to school rather than letting me drive her there, even when it was raining.

But I never thought anything was particularly wrong; I just assumed it was part of normal adolescence. I'd been very sporty at her age and very thin. In fact I was so thin I remember eating to try and put on weight. So, really, what I was seeing was my daughter doing similar things to what I had done at her age. I thought all the healthy eating and exercising was... well... healthy.

What I did notice, however, was that she was horrified when she began her periods. She could not cope with having a period; she hated it. But, again, I just thought this was normal teenage girl stuff.

Then she became obsessed with cooking. She'd read and read cookbooks, and collect them, so much so that her schoolteachers asked me if she was thinking of a career as a dietician or a chef. We had stacks of recipe books everywhere, piled up on the coffee table and the floor. It drove me mad sometimes!

Then, around six months before her 15th birthday, she came to me and said: "Mummy, I haven't grown since March and I haven't had a period in two months."

So I checked her height, as I recorded her height every few months on the kitchen door as well as that of her younger sister. This was the first summer that she hadn't grown at all. I thought this was a bit odd. But I wasn't too alarmed about the periods because my own periods had been quite erratic when I was her age. What did worry me, though, was the fact that she was drinking copious amounts of water. All the family noticed it, but again this was something that I'd done when I was her age. Nevertheless, I didn't think it would be a bad thing to run it all in front of the GP. So we went along to the doctors' surgery.

The GP felt Lauren should be checked for diabetes. She asked me a few questions related to symptoms of diabetes and I said, "Yes, yes, yes, that's going on" and so on. Lauren had the usual blood tests. But they came back as inconclusive. She didn't have diabetes.

So I took her back to the GP who wondered if it might be a urinary tract infection. "But she hasn't got a temperature," I said. But I thought, well okay, she's the doctor, she's the expert so she must know.

Again the results came back as inconclusive. So back we went again and this time the GP said that it was probably "just a bit of a phase" that my daughter was going through. She asked us to come back in a few months to check on how things were going.

So I thought well, okay, fine… The GP did ask me if Lauren was eating and I said, "Oh yes, there are no problems there!" Because you have to understand that she *was* eating at this stage. In fact she seemed to be eating just fine. We always sat down at the dinner table and ate together as a family, none of this eating in front of the TV stuff. And of course whenever I took her back home to Australia there would be our extended family, all 11 or 12 of them, sitting around the table, eating together. But little did I know that, afterwards, Lauren was purging her calories out through exercise. I never thought to mention the exercising to the GP; remember at this stage I thought it was normal.

We spent that Christmas in Australia. Everyone in my family noticed the unusual amount of water that Lauren was drinking and we all tried to intervene. But nobody actually noticed that she was underweight. All I can think of is that she managed to hide it really well. Basically, I think she would eat and eat and eat whatever she wanted and then exercise like crazy to get rid of it.

Back in the UK, I remember noticing her weighing out fruit on a couple of occasions and even measuring the size of a banana. When I quizzed her about it she said she was just sorting out her five a day. So, again, I didn't think anything of it.

Then at Easter she went off on holiday for a fortnight with her father and stepmother. She came back on a Sunday night. I'd saved some of our roast dinner for her, but she hardly ate a thing. I assumed it must be because she'd had a big lunch with her dad, so I left it at that.

The next morning she didn't have any breakfast which I thought was strange. Then, the next day, I got a call from the school nurse who said, "I don't think Lauren's very well". She suggested I take her back to the GP, so off we went again.

This time it was a different GP and she seemed to really know her stuff. The GP weighed her and checked out the previous weights on Lauren's notes. I could see the GP was worried. Lauren had been asked to strip down to her underwear to be weighed. For months I'd only seen her in baggy clothes and, of course, she'd been away from me for a fortnight with her dad. This was the first time I'd seen just how thin she'd become and I was horrified. Lauren was diagnosed with anorexia and referred to the local specialist eating disorders service. But they couldn't take her for six weeks or so. Still reeling from the diagnosis and seeing Lauren looking so painfully thin, I panicked. What was I supposed to do in these six weeks? All I knew was that I just had to get Lauren to eat.

The first thing I did was to take her to our favourite restaurant up the road, thinking that she'd love that. But of course she couldn't eat anything. By this stage I had no idea what I was up against, so I just kept trying to get her to eat. But she refused everything.

I sent her to school and asked the teachers and the nurse to ensure she ate her lunch, explaining that she'd been diagnosed with anorexia. But somehow, unbeknown to me, she managed to avoid having lunch. By this time I was beginning to seriously worry. I called eating disorder helplines, counsellors, psychologists and anyone who claimed to treat eating disorders just to work out the best course of action. I scoured the internet, wondering what I should do. I came across websites that gave some pretty horrific "causes" of eating disorders. One website suggested that anorexia was a result of being sexually abused as a child. Well, my imagination began to run riot. I was dismayed!

A week went by and Lauren came back from a school outing. It was 11.30 at night. As soon as she got off the bus I could see that this was pretty serious. She was listless; it was as if the life had been completely sucked out of her. She'd eaten hardly anything at all in a week, despite my efforts to get her to eat.

I immediately took her to A&E where they gave her 500ml of glucose. The people at the hospital were very good, actually, except for the admitting nurse who asked her why on earth couldn't she eat? What was wrong with her? What was I - her mother - doing to *prevent* her from eating? That kind of thing... I'll never forget the way that nurse looked at me. But to be honest I didn't really care. I just felt enormous relief. I thought, "It's going to be okay. We're in a hospital now. They'll be able to fix this".

They checked Lauren's pulse rate and blood sugar, both of which were very low. The glucose helped to bring them back up again, only to come crashing back down. The nurse said that we couldn't give her any more glucose. She'd need to have something else like an energy drink, an apple juice or something. She was admitted to the paediatric ward for observation where they promised they'd try and get her to eat breakfast when the time came.

It was 1 o'clock in the morning by then and I sat with her the whole time. Lauren did drink some of the energy drink they'd given her which helped a little. At daybreak, I suddenly realised my younger daughter would be waiting to be taken to school. So I went home, sorted her out and came back to the hospital where I was told that Lauren had eaten a bowl of cereal, some juice and a banana. They said she'd done really well. I was delighted. I was told that the consultant paediatrician and an eating disorders nurse would be coming to see us.

The eating disorders nurse spent about an hour-and-a-half with us. She talked to us about the dangers of anorexia, what it does to your organs, how the fat around the organs which is there to protect them disappears and how the body is living off the fat of the organs rather than the fat of the food you are giving your body. She also explained what happens to your bones and so on. The whole lot.

It scared Lauren and it scared me even more. This nurse also showed me how to feed her and how to put a meal plan together. It was based on portion sizes and not calories, initially half portions increasing over time. And she was to have three meals and three snacks a day. Also, Lauren was to be banned from the kitchen so she couldn't hover around watching me cook. Most important of all, I had to get her to eat.

My response was, "Okay, this sounds easy enough to do". Little did I know… An appointment was fixed for a few days' time for an assessment with the consultant psychiatrist from the specialist eating disorders service. So I took Lauren home and began to feed her.

She protested heavily, but we sat down three times a day for meals and I made sure she had three snacks a day. She managed okay, but there was a lot of anxiety and a lot of head banging and self-harm and food throwing. She said she wanted to kill herself, she wanted to die. She would run around the house, up and down the stairs. I knew I had to take drastic measures. So I took her out of school and adopted the "life stops until you eat" approach. No exercise, no school, no running up and down the stairs constantly; our lives were consumed by the meal plan.

I had to remove all sharp objects that she might have access to. She often confined herself to her room. She would scream, she would howl, she would bang her head and pull her hair out, none of which I knew how to deal with. Each day we just lived hour by hour.

I couldn't go to the supermarket without her being glued to my hip. Everything was scrutinised. She read every label. She was a walking encyclopaedia of calorie and fat content and nutritional information. It was very frustrating but somehow I did get her to eat the three meals and three snacks a day. But it was sheer hell because every time we sat down it was a struggle.

We eventually met with the specialist eating disorders service. They set us up with weekly appointments. Lauren would be weighed and measured every week. They also gave us a list from which she had to choose breakfast, snacks and so on. Meanwhile, I kept a diary of what she ate every day and it worked. She did it. But not without a lot of anxiety.

She went through a purging phase where she'd eat and then throw up. It was one of her friends who told me that she'd heard Lauren in the bathroom trying to throw up after we'd had dinner and I put a stop to that immediately. Her keyworker told me to go with her to the bathroom after meals and sit outside with the door open. We went through this routine for about four months. I was actually very grateful for this advice because it worked and stopped the purging dead in its tracks!

I'll never forget the occasion when Lauren was told by her keyworker that she'd have to increase from half portions to three-quarter portions in her meal plan. Before I could stop her she shot out of the clinic and literally threw herself into the road, right in front of the oncoming traffic. A truck driver slammed on the brakes and stopped in time. I went hysterical! I dragged Lauren back into the clinic where I continued to be hysterical only to be told: "Pull yourself together, Mrs Dawson. If Lauren had really wanted to kill herself then she would have done so. We feel she's fine."

So from that moment on I knew I was pretty much on my own.

Thankfully it was around this time that I came across the F.E.A.S.T. website and the Around The Dinner Table forum. Actually it was one of the mums at school who told me about it. So I went onto the website where I found a link to the book *Help Your Teenager Beat an Eating Disorder* by David Lock & Daniel Le Grange. From the moment it arrived in the post, everything just seemed to fall into place. Becoming well-read around this subject was the most important action I could take, and as soon as I learned that anorexia is a biological brain-based illness, I just "got it". After that, I really went to town. I read everything I could get my hands on regarding the biological nature of this illness.

One day Lauren came to me in the kitchen. She was distraught. She said: "What is happening to me? Will it ever go away? How did it start?" So I suggested we sit down and have a think. I pointed out the obsession with healthy eating, the exercising, the stockpiling of cookbooks... And she said: "You know what? That started even earlier, much earlier, right back in year 8" and that's when she proceeded to tell me more about the way she'd begun to adhere to all these "healthy eating" and "five a day" messages like glue. "Mum, it got to the stage where I'd even exercise away a piece of toast!" she explained.

Anyway, I knew I had to get my daughter well. And to begin with, I had to get the weight back onto her. Over the next few months I watched her weight like a hawk. I also did what a lot of families do, I guess, and sneak high calorie ingredients into things in a bid to put on the weight: a slug of double cream into the soup, extra oil into the curry and so forth.

After a hellish January with Lauren raging, yelling and head banging virtually every night, these distressing behaviours suddenly came to a stop. Completely out of the blue, just like that. I'd been reading about how the brain needs fats; indeed I'd read that more than half of the brain consists of fat and cholesterol.

Well, I'd been slipping all these extra fats into our meals and I wondered whether that was anything to do with Lauren's change of behaviour. That, plus the fact that she was finally getting a nutritionally balanced diet.

Things continued to improve. In the summer we went out to Australia for a big family reunion. Lauren was just beginning to put on a little bit of weight. My family took over and did her meals and snacks in shifts to give me a break. Being with all her cousins and being around the big family dinner table three times a day really made a difference to her and she started eating. There was very rarely a complaint apart from the occasional snack that she couldn't manage. But for the most part she kept her cool. She even started to eat puddings. I remember going out to a restaurant and Lauren ordering a huge meal and a massive pudding with ice cream. I exchanged glances with the rest of the family as if to say: "Oh my God!" It really was amazing, because she ate everything she was served up.

I was still trying to sneak high calorie stuff into the meals on occasions. I'd ask my sister to do it, too, when she was cooking. Lauren would never question what anyone else cooked, only what I cooked and so she'd eat it. By now I was becoming the Bad Guy. One day she caught me adding cream to a sauce. After that she wouldn't trust me.

But while we were away for all that time in Australia she put on quite a few kilos. Back in the UK school started again. But Lauren couldn't eat her lunch or snacks in front of her peers. So we got into a routine whereby she'd have a reasonable breakfast. Then I'd go into school in the middle of the morning and sit with her in the car while she had her snack. I'd bring her home for lunch and then take her back to school for the afternoon.

I remember the day her periods began again, six months from the date of diagnosis. I was thrilled. I went out and bought her a beautiful gold bracelet which I knew she really wanted. I told her how proud I was of her because she'd worked so hard.

Another motivator on the weight-gain front was a school trip, planned for after Christmas. We all agreed that unless she reached a certain weight target, then she wouldn't be allowed to go. She worked really, really hard to gain that weight, and she succeeded. It was funny, because the dietician and I worked out an entire meal plan for her to take with her on that trip. So that's the way it was at that point and she did really well.

By Easter Lauren was able to start eating lunch at school with her friends. She was also able to manage her own snacks, albeit in private. By May she was fully weight restored at a healthy weight which she managed to maintain - and then in the July she was discharged from treatment. The psychiatrist insisted she was fully recovered. And that was that. We were suddenly set adrift on our own without any form of after-care support. Because she was weight restored it was assumed that she was well. But she was far from well. I noticed a number of behaviours which suggested she wasn't coping as well as she should have been, given her age. So we kind of muddled through the summer. Also, shortly before she was discharged from treatment I became the enemy. And I still am. She won't talk to me unless she needs money or a lift or something. I'm the arch-baddie and I really don't know why.

Recently I had a chat with a leading eating disorders expert. I told him about all the anger that was going on in Lauren's life and the way much of it seemed to be directed at me. The good news was that he confirmed that, yes, Lauren was fully recovered from the eating disorder. But he also explained that anger can be part of the process of recovery; indeed he said that it can indicate a strong recovery. So I am hoping that, before long, the anger will subside and we can become close again, just like we used to be before the illness struck.

Despite the rift between Lauren and me, our story does show that there is light at the end of the tunnel. But it's been a punishingly tough ride.

I attribute a large part of Lauren's recovery to her sheer grit and determination. For instance she really wanted to go on that school trip I mentioned earlier and knew that if she didn't put on weight then she couldn't go. So she got stuck in and got the weight on. She worked really hard and she did it.

After that, whenever there was something she wanted to achieve or do, it would motivate her to keep working on her recovery. For example she really wanted to be able to eat lunch at school with the other kids. So she worked on it and did this, too.

There was always a carrot in front of her and, once she was able to do something without feeling anxious about it, we'd move on to the next thing, and then the next, and the next. And slowly but surely her brain became fully restored. So much so that some five months after that school trip she was doing everything on her own. We went into a totally normal existence.

But you know what? Not once during our time at the eating disorder service did I ever hear much emphasis on: "You've got to get the weight on first and foremost before you do anything else."

I found this really strange. But it didn't stop me from following the advice in all those books I'd read and which I'd found on the F.E.A.S.T. website and ATDT forum. From the time of diagnosis until probably Easter 2012 I fed my child with three meals and three snacks a day. After Easter we relaxed a little and cut out the evening snack. But, throughout, my focus was on getting one-hundred-per-cent nutrition into my daughter one-hundred-per-cent of the time. No ifs, no buts - life stopped until Lauren was gaining weight regularly and had got into the habit of eating normally.

I am convinced that this approach made a huge, huge difference to her recovery and why she was weight restored in just six months rather than 18 months, two years, three years or even longer.

I have reached the stage where I've promised Lauren that I won't talk about eating disorders unless there's a need. She wants to put all this behind her, and I can get on with my life, too. Only yesterday I was driving home from work and felt strangely calm for the first time in two years. It was really weird because I suddenly thought: "I can think of something else now. I can do something new. I can apply for that job I've always wanted, go on holiday, whatever." As I sat in the rush hour traffic I thought: "This is good, really good."

I am literally moving on for the first time in two years. As for the rift between Lauren and myself, I am hoping that it will eventually heal - sooner rather than later. And I'll make sure she knows that I'm always here for her should she need me.

After all, that's what mums are for.

Kathleen's story

"I can't tell you how desperate we were for someone to come and talk to us about the illness - to explain what we could expect, what was normal and what wasn't. We kept waiting. But there seemed to be nobody."

I'd always been one to read articles on medical and health issues, but never anorexia. Just a glance at those awful pictures would make me want to turn the page straight away. And, anyway, anorexia happened to other families, didn't it? Families obsessed with diets, picky eaters, "pushy" parents and so on. Not to happy, healthy families like ours.

So, when our only child Freya began to show signs of an eating disorder at around the age of 12, I think this perception kept us in a kind of denial. We found ourselves explaining away some of the signs that we might otherwise have picked up on simply because we just never expected our daughter to get anorexia.

My husband Martin and I first realised there was a problem in September 2011. But, looking back, there were many, many signs before then. I even wonder if Freya's problems stem back as far as primary school, when her best friend moved to another part of the country and she was left alone. At the age of seven or eight I remember her having thoughts about "not deserving" food, mainly things like chocolate and crisps. But it didn't set off any alarm bells because, like most families, we were totally ignorant of the illness.

Martin and I are both tall and slim, the kind of people who could eat anything without putting on any weight. In our family there was never any talk of dieting. We ate most meals together at the table and food was always a pleasure. We didn't even own any bathroom weighing scales. I mean, why on earth would we?

Then, during the first year at senior school in 2010/11, Freya started seriously restricting her food intake and we noticed that she was getting thinner. She'd begun to go through puberty the previous Christmas and was starting to look more like a young woman than a little girl. But by the beginning of year 8 it was as if she'd gone backwards again. Four of her cousins had gone through a skinny phase at the start of puberty, so at first we explained this away.

We also noticed a change in Freya's behaviour. She became very controlling, determined to get her own way. We thought this odd because, all through her childhood, she'd had a very sunny, easy-going disposition and would nearly always do as she was asked. We put it down to "becoming a teenager".

The first concern came in the summer of 2011. Freya came back from a short holiday with her grandparents. They told us that she had eaten very little. But we didn't worry too much as she was eating perfectly normally at home at this point - or so we thought!

Freya had always been an early riser and so, during the 2011 summer holidays, we'd been allowing her to get her own cereal in the mornings. By September we realised that the cereal box wasn't getting lighter each day. I could hear her pouring the cereal into the bowl but what I didn't hear was her carefully spooning most of it back into the box again!

Each evening as I cooked supper Freya would suddenly appear at my side and watch my every move like a hawk. When it was time to dish up the meal she would say: "Don't give me much because I'm not very hungry." She would then wolf down her meal as if she were starving. We later found out that she'd been throwing away her packed lunch at school - this, on top of the tiny amount of cereal she'd had for breakfast. The evening meal was the only decent portion of food she was eating throughout the day. No wonder she was wolfing it down!

At first we thought Freya was skipping meals in order to "fit in" with the popular crowd at school. The "cool girls" were all really slim and she wanted to be like them. But, of course, we thought we'd be able to talk her out of this and make her see sense. But as autumn went on, we began to realise that things were out of her control. Her fear of eating was so intense that she could not overcome it.

By this point, Martin and I were getting very anxious. We had no knowledge of the illness nor how to deal with it. And there was still an element of denial; we couldn't believe this was happening to our lovely girl.

From this point onwards, Freya deteriorated very quickly. It was terrifying to watch especially as she'd always been very slim. Also, because she hadn't fully gone through puberty, there was very little weight to lose before things became serious. Worse, once her emerging eating disorder was out in the open, she felt she no longer had to hide things from us and pretend that everything was okay. As a result she began to eat less and less.

We took Freya to see our GP in the October half-term break. We knew by this stage that she was seriously ill, that it was probably an eating disorder and that Freya needed urgent help. The thing is, as a family we rarely went to the GP. Freya had always been a really healthy child. Indeed we'd only needed to take her once or twice since toddlerhood.

We assumed the GP would explain all about eating disorders and talk us through the referral process for treatment. In the event we just had the usual quick ten minutes during which time the GP said very little.

I think at that stage I was in such a state myself that I didn't know what questions to ask. I panicked and my mind went completely blank. Martin and I knew there was a serious problem and we were really scared of what this would mean for Freya. It was only afterwards when we came away that we wished we'd said more.

I did manage to explain that Freya had become extremely anxious around food and that, by this stage, she was eating about a third of her normal diet. The GP listened and said that he would refer her to CAMHS. He told Freya to eat as much as she could while waiting for the appointment to come through. But the GP didn't weigh her or measure her height. If he had then he might have noticed that her BMI was dangerously low. But of course Martin and I still hadn't a clue what we were dealing with so we had no concept of dangerously low BMIs. We didn't even know what Freya weighed, or should weigh, because children aren't routinely weighed here in the UK. I think the last time she'd been weighed was when she was a baby!

The GP didn't talk to us about eating disorders. Nor did he check her blood pressure or pulse. But at least he agreed to refer her to CAMHS, which helped to put our minds at rest.

Of course we had no idea how long it would take for the CAMHS appointment to come through. In the meantime things took a turn for the worse. Because her eating disorder was now out in the open, Freya found it easier than ever to cut back. When we took her to the GP we knew it was serious, but we didn't know how quickly we would need to react or how quickly things would go downhill from then.

A week after the GP's appointment, we went to a friend's birthday party. Freya promised she would eat some food, but when it came to it she just couldn't. I will never forget the look of terror on her face as she surveyed the table of party food. She'd been outside to visit the family's rabbits and when she came back indoors she was frozen. She just couldn't get warm again. When we got home we insisted that she had something to eat. Martin and I sat with her for two long hours during which time we only managed to get her to eat half an apple and a few sips of milk. By now we were terrified.

That weekend she ate next to nothing and, as I watched her leave for school on the Monday morning, I knew that she wouldn't last the day. I went online to see what help I could find, and came across the Beat website - the UK eating disorders charity. I phoned their helpline and sobbed down the phone to the lovely lady on the other end. She told me that I would have to "jump up and down" to get help for my child. In the weeks that followed her words would haunt me.

The moment I put down the phone, the school called to say Freya was feeling unwell and could I come and pick her up. Then, on the way to school, her form tutor phoned to say she had concerns about Freya and could she meet with me when I got to school. I explained that we had recently discovered that Freya had an eating disorder. She called the Head of Year who immediately came to join us. Both teachers urged me to take Freya to A&E and demand help.

Martin and I rushed her over to A&E that afternoon. She was already very thin and we were worried that if she lost more weight we would be heading for really critical territory. After a long wait she was examined by a doctor. They did all the appropriate tests and checked her heart and blood pressure, and took blood samples. Her weight was very low. Her heart was checked and thankfully that was okay. Freya was admitted to the paediatric ward. We spent four days there during which time her blood pressure and blood sugar were checked every four hours. Both were very low. By this stage she was eating next to nothing. But, during the whole stay, we never got to see a doctor or a psychiatrist. I was in too much of a state to start "jumping up and down" at this stage. I was paralysed with fear.

We could see that, physically, Freya was very weak. But nobody came and tried to help in any way - to get her to eat, talk to her about the situation she was in or explain what needed to happen. I was trying to get her to eat little bits and pieces throughout the day but she just got hysterical. We were very conscious that, all around us, there were some very sick children and we didn't want to provoke this hysterical reaction in Freya because it would disturb the others.

It was the most awful, awful time. Freya was terrified, too. She just couldn't eat and was really frightened of where she was and what was going on. She simply didn't understand what was happening to her. Neither did we.

I can't tell you how desperate we were for someone to come along and talk to us about the illness, explain what we could expect, and

what was normal and what wasn't. We kept waiting for somebody...
I mean, whenever your child is ill you always think there's going to be
somebody, maybe a doctor or someone else that can step in and help.
But there seemed to be nobody. It was terrifying.

After four days in hospital a doctor came to see us and said Freya
was being discharged into the care of CAMHS and she was to see
them later that afternoon. So we thought: "Phew! This is where she
gets treatment. This is where we find out what's going on and how
we can help." We finally had a ray of hope.

We took her along to the appointment where Freya was assessed
by a CAMHS nurse. We explained that she wasn't eating and that we
needed urgent help. But it was all about assessing and form filling.
And so nothing happened. It was the worst thing in the world,
having been in hospital where we had the reassurance that our
daughter was being checked and monitored constantly, to be
despatched off home with a very sick and frail child. Suddenly it hit
us - the realisation that we were going to have to soldier on at home,
on our own, without any medical checks. What if her condition
deteriorated? Without the heart and blood checks, we simply
wouldn't know! It really was so very frightening.

Thankfully we had a second appointment with CAMHS the
following week, and we assumed this would be the start of treatment.
But when we returned, we just carried on filling out forms and
signing things. "Okay," we thought, "I guess this kind of thing has to
be done. Now for the actual treatment itself..." We waited for the
nurse to set a further appointment, this time with a psychiatrist, only
to be told that an appointment would "come through in the post in
the near future".

I thought, "Oh my goodness, nothing's going to happen!" It was
just total shock and horror, really, that we were in this awful, awful
place and they weren't going to help us straight away. The nurse said
that in the meantime she would phone me every couple of days to see
how things were.

So we went home. By now we were desperate. But I thought,

"Well at least the CAMHS nurse is going to phone me regularly, at least that's something." If things got worse there would be someone to talk to. The nurse phoned me the next day with details of the Beat helpline, which I'd already found, and then I never heard from her again.

Every time I tried to phone CAMHS to find out about our appointment, I got an answer machine. Or I got a secretary who couldn't put me through to anyone. The sense of isolation and fear, and of not knowing where to go for help, was truly dreadful.

Three days later a letter arrived with an appointment to see the psychiatrist... in three weeks' time. We knew that if we didn't get Freya to eat soon she wouldn't be alive to meet the psychiatrist. By this time a single day was like a month. I was desperately trying to get her to eat and drink. Meanwhile I could see her getting more and more frail in front of my eyes. But I just didn't know what to do because, at that stage, I knew that if I pushed her she'd get hysterical. I worried it was doing more damage than good.

It was during those three weeks that I began to take Beat up on their advice and start "jumping up and down". Martin and I decided we couldn't wait any longer. I started to phone round everyone. I called the hospital and the GP (who told us about an adult eating disorders unit, who said they couldn't help). CAMHS couldn't help, either. They wouldn't let us come in sooner. It seemed that whichever way I turned I was faced with a brick wall. There was nobody that could offer any help. All anyone did was to refer us back to CAMHS; CAMHS would be the people who would help us. The thing is I just couldn't get through to CAMHS. Time after time I'd get that confounded answer machine. And on the few occasions when I did manage to get through to the secretary it was all "No, sorry, the psychiatrist doesn't have any appointments sooner".

It didn't seem to matter how desperate the situation was. All I seemed to get was: "We can't help you, sorry." They simply said that if we had any concerns about Freya's physical health then we should take her back to A&E, which, no doubt would mean her being admitted to the paediatric ward again where nothing would happen. It was like nightmarish revolving doors that led nowhere. And this was our beautiful daughter's life that was at stake!

At this stage Martin even said: "Perhaps no-one will help us because they think we are bad parents." We honestly thought at that time that the medical professionals were prepared to let our daughter die. That's how desperate our thought processes had got by then.

We had absolutely no support. We were on our own and terrified. And we were so very, very tired. I mean, we weren't sleeping. We were up every hour or so, checking that Freya's heart hadn't stopped during the night. It was that bad.

I phoned the Beat helpline a few times. I also spoke to a friend of a friend whose daughter had recovered from anorexia. This lady's daughter had spent three months in an eating disorders unit. She had been referred when her parents refused to leave A&E until they saw a psychiatrist. For the first time we had to face the awful possibility that Freya might have to be admitted to an eating disorders unit.

At this point we decided to try a private therapist. We took Freya to see a hypnotherapist in the run up to Christmas. Amazingly the hypnotherapist seemed to get through to Freya, possibly because she told her from the word go that she would speak to her as if she were an adult and not a child. From that first meeting Freya accepted that she needed to increase her food intake and, although it was torture for her, she agreed to increase what she ate by a little each day. It was painfully slow progress but at least it was a start in the right direction.

However, not long afterwards, we had to take Freya back to A&E as we were concerned there might be a problem with her kidneys.

After a long wait, tests revealed that her kidneys were fine. But when they weighed her they discovered she'd lost even more weight. They were very concerned. They talked to us about her mental state and they talked to Freya, too.

It was the first time we'd heard her talk about suicide, self-harming and thoughts of running away. We had no idea she was thinking things like this. Okay she'd get hysterical whenever we tried to get her to eat but there was no hint of any of this.

The hospital offered to admit her but, because it was the weekend, there was no psychiatrist on duty. So we took her home again because at least we were able to get her to eat at home. We were concerned that she might have been too traumatised to eat in hospital.

Then, just before Christmas, we got our long-awaited appointment with the psychiatrist who told us that Freya would need to be assessed at the local eating disorders unit as her weight was dangerously low.

At that point, because she was eating a little bit more every day, we began to wonder if we could get her well at home instead. And, with the threat of hospitalisation hanging over her, Freya tried her very best to increase her food intake. So, when the letter came through from the unit asking us to bring her in for an assessment, it was really hard for us. We'd never entertained the thought that she would have to go into a unit.

But, at the assessment, it was made clear to us that Freya's life was in danger at such a low weight. So, despite the progress she had managed to make at home, we agreed to have her admitted immediately. We were devastated. I think I accepted it more than Martin. I think he thought that if we just kept going then we could do this at home. But I was completely exhausted by this stage.

In the event things actually got worse after Freya was admitted. At home we'd got her up to half portions of food which, looking back on what was going on at the time, was amazing. But when they took her into the unit she managed to persuade them that she was only on quarter portions. So they started her off on very small portions. As a result she lost a further kilo.

Freya spent eight months in the unit. She had a lot of weight to gain, so it was a long haul. However she complied with the programme. They aimed for a kilo a week and, most weeks, she succeeded. Underneath the anorexia, Freya was a very conforming child. She would always do whatever she was asked. She was never one to draw attention to herself or make a fuss. This is why the illness was so shocking because her personality transformed completely.

But it also meant that she did what she was asked in the unit, although I think the main reason she did so was because she felt that the sooner she arrived at her target weight the sooner she could come back home and lose it all again. And the more she interacted with the other young people in the unit, all of whom were older than her, the more bad habits and tricks she picked up. They'd swap tips and try out the same things. It was all about trying to get one over the staff all the time, hiding food and exercising in secret.

Freya was discharged in the summer. She'd gone into the unit as a little girl but emerged as a sassy teenager. Her mental state had deteriorated, she was self-harming and we began to experience rage and abuse which she had never shown at home. So bringing her home wasn't the joyful occasion it should have been because we knew that we were bringing home a very sick girl.

Freya went back under the care of CAMHS, and saw a psychiatrist each week to be weighed. She also had appointments with a psychologist and a family therapy team. She'd try and hoodwink her psychiatrist who would ask her if she was hiding weights, had drunk a load of water or whatever. The psychiatrist obviously knew about the tricks, but she didn't seem overly worried about them. We were saying: "Look she's pushing us back on the amount of calories she's having every day. She's not having enough." And the psychiatrist would respond with: "Oh, but her weight's showing that she's still in a safe range, it's okay."

But when eventually we realised that it wasn't okay and that she'd been water-loading we were back in that dangerous place again. As parents we could see all this happening at home but it's almost as if the clinicians were listening to Freya rather than listening to us. So we ended up back in the dangerous place very quickly. I think that if they'd talked to us more and listened to what we had to say then they could have helped us put the brakes on it, put the frighteners on

Freya a bit and get her back into hospital to be reassessed sooner.

At home we were struggling to cope. There were constant rages and self-harming; we'd even had to pull her in off the roof on one occasion. She would frequently bang her head against the walls which left her forehead bruised and sore. Once you've lived through this kind of thing for a few weeks and then a few months you quickly get to the point where you can't cope any longer. We were unable to get through to Freya, and by the autumn she'd lost enough weight to be reassessed at the unit. We felt it was inevitable that she would go back in.

In the event Freya wasn't readmitted to the unit. Instead they gave her two weeks during which time they said that her behaviour needed to improve and she needed to increase her intake of food, back to gaining a kilo a month, or she'd be readmitted. And so we came home.

Martin and I weren't very optimistic. We felt that the illness would suck her further and further down. But we were wrong. Freya complied and succeeded in turning things around. The aggression and abuse gradually faded and she managed to take control of her feelings more. She also began to accept that she needed to eat more. And so it was a gradual process from then onwards. It was all really down to us within the family to get her to eat enough to gain weight. We didn't have much external support.

While Freya was in the unit we were taught how to manage meal times, but if a child is determined not to eat there is a limit to what can be achieved. In the end it was the threat of going back into hospital that made Freya decide to work with us.

As parents, we didn't have any emotional support. Thankfully another mum at the hospital had recommended the F.E.A.S.T. website and the Around The Dinner Table forum. These resources saved my life really. When I went onto the forum and read about the rage and abuse that everyone around the world was experiencing, I suddenly realised that this was a "normal" feature of the illness. I was just so relieved, because I'd thought: "Is something else wrong? Is there another dimension to her illness?" But, no, I learned that all of this was part of the process, for so many families. Knowing that our case wasn't unusual really helped me. Also, reading about how other families were coping and dealing with the illness helped us to cope better. It had a huge impact, especially on my ability to cope as a mother.

It took three months for Freya to steadily increase her intake. By the New Year we'd managed to get her calories up to a higher level. She's just about managed to gain her kilo a month since then. So, for us, that's been a huge bonus. When we think where we were only a few months ago... but we still have a long way to go. We're going to be working on the weight for the rest of the year. So we battle on, rejoicing in every small bit of progress.

Freya has been at school full-time since September. We have used this as leverage, telling her that we'd have to take her out of school if her weight begins to fall again. She loves school, so that's been a good motivator.

We've also introduced other caveats. For example she loves swimming and she's not allowed to swim until she gets up to her target weight. She still finds it hard to go it alone; she looks to us for all the support. But at least, thanks to resources like the forum, we know what we're supposed to be doing.

As her mother and somebody who is with her most of the time, I know that she's making progress. But it's little things that maybe only a mum would notice. I'm not convinced that CAMHS are noticing these. They're asking her to "challenge the eating disorder" and telling us that we're not "challenging" it enough. But, to me, the little things are her gradual way of doing this - she can't take massive steps all at once.

I believe that, unless you live with the illness day after day like a parent does, you wouldn't be aware of these very subtle yet positive changes. There have been a couple of major things. For example the period just before evening meals tends to be her most anxious time and I've learned that the best way to react is to say very little and give her a hug which is usually enough to calm her down and help her to cope with the anxiety. We just talk about it passing.

I don't always manage to keep calm, though... For example, a few weeks ago she'd been quite difficult. My tone changed and I was quite assertive with her about her behaviour and she said: "Mum, don't get angry with me because the eating disorder voice is shouting at me and I don't want you to shout at me as well; I want you to be calm." It was the first time that she'd separated herself from the illness.

When I look back there's been a definite shift. Before it was a case of her eating "just enough" so she didn't have to go back into hospital, but already I'm noticing the distinct green shoots of her working with us towards recovery. It's hard to pinpoint when the change took place. It was a very subtle shift. Of course I know we still have a long way to go and I'm not naïve enough to think that it will be a straight path without any glitches.

One of the things that I believe helped to turn things around is knowledge: as parents knowing what to do and how to do it, learning how to cope with the illness and how to guide your child towards recovery. The trouble is, as far as treatment teams are concerned, I'm not convinced that parents are valued in the way they should be as a vital part of the mix. We need to be coached and trained. We also need emotional support. I often find myself being a counsellor, psychologist, dietician and a mum, all at the same time, but I don't have training in any of this aside from what I've learned through books, researching online, contacting parents of other sufferers, visiting the ATDT forum and looking through the F.E.A.S.T. resources.

Back at the start I wish I'd known what signs to look out for - and also the fact that there is a level of deception that comes with the illness that makes these hard to spot. If I'd known more back then I believe I would have been in a far better position to fight for treatment for my daughter.

Both Martin and I feel guilty that we didn't pick up on Freya's eating disorder sooner, even though I have no idea how we would have done so because we knew nothing about the signs. And, as I said earlier, you just don't expect this kind of thing to happen to your family.

There is so much conflicting advice out there, but I am learning to trust my intuition as a parent. No-one knows my child as well as me. I've come to realise that, sometimes, the experts can be grappling around in the dark as much as I am. However, I have one advantage over them in that I will never give up on my daughter. There is no love like a mother's love for her child and that is my most powerful weapon against Freya's anorexia.

MY TIPS:

Visit the F.E.A.S.T. website and ATDT forum - both are outstanding resources for parents. (See list of resources at the end of the book.)

Read and research as much as you can. (See list of resources at the end of the book.)

Don't automatically assume that GPs and other medical practitioners will have an extensive knowledge of eating disorders.

Be assertive in securing help for your child - you may have to fight to get the care you need for your child. Also, be prepared to be the leader in your child's treatment team.

Don't accept that medical professionals know what is best for your child - if you are caring for your child at home you will learn what works and what doesn't. Practical experience can often count for more than theories.

Trust your instincts as a parent.

Look after yourself - battling with an eating disorder is a long and difficult fight. If you get to the stage where you're finding it hard to cope, please do seek help for yourself.

Don't expect family and friends to understand what you are going through. Seek out other parents in the same situation and support each other.

Eating disorders can be overcome - don't ever lose hope.

Elaine's story

"With someone like Lydia who doesn't handle change well, continuity is vital. But, at 18, patients are cut adrift from the treatment team they've come to know and trust to face the mysterious new world of Adult Services."

My daughter, Lydia, had a history of obsessive behaviours - for example her teachers would remark on the way she'd constantly wash her hands at school. She was also fussy and stubborn as a child, and extremely anxious. Then, when she was 13 or 14, she began to lose weight. By the spring of 2009 I was beginning to worry that she could be developing an eating disorder. She later told me that it had probably been germinating for 12 months or so, completely undetected by any of us.

Lydia wasn't just losing weight; she was isolating herself and being aggressive. Certain situations had always made her anxious. Travelling, for example, was something that was getting worse at this time. She would always have some kind of outburst a day or so before going on holiday and during travelling. She'd kick off at the airport and I'm sure everyone must have thought I was a terrible mother who couldn't discipline my child. Gradually, her obsessive behaviours got worse and worse with the result that, eventually, it was difficult to take her away on holiday at all.

Lydia would refuse to go out anywhere. She also hated going anywhere near sand, so holidays at the seaside were out. She'd lock herself in the bathroom. Also, it was impossible to find her something to eat as she'd always been extremely fussy over food. But increasingly she'd run away, jump out of the car at traffic lights, even hit out at me - the anxiety was so strong.

Meanwhile I was getting more and more anxious, too. I was also feeling very helpless and, if the truth be told, I was in a kind of denial. I just wished that whatever "it" was would just go away. But of course "it" didn't and by the age of 15 Lydia's weight had dropped to quite a low point. But it was all so very gradual at this stage, beginning with the obsessive behaviours and followed by the desire to lose weight.

Time and time again, I'd wonder why this was happening. Had we done something wrong? Was there something going on elsewhere? I knew she was unhappy at school. She'd had a long history of trouble with her teachers at primary school. Lydia was impulsive and couldn't sit still. She was also stubborn and defiant. Her teachers reacted so negatively that she lost her confidence and began to withdraw from her friends and become extremely shy.

At home she was difficult to handle. She was stubborn, wanted a lot of attention, had difficulty seeing another person's point of view and seemed to have little awareness of other people's needs. She continued to lock herself in the bathroom and refused to participate in family outings or other activities like watching the TV - all kinds of things. She wouldn't even look at her baby brother let alone touch him. In fact she was negative and aggressive towards her siblings in general.

Whenever we took her to see a medical professional they'd always be looking for some fault in the family. They'd accuse us of being over-anxious and of having tensions in the family. But, to be honest, what family wouldn't be anxious or tense if their child had been behaving in this way for years and years?

Lydia would vent all her frustrations at home, so we took the brunt of everything. We were her "punch bag", if you like, and she'd take it all out on us - the fact that she felt unable to fit in at school and was so painfully shy and, presumably, lonely. The result was unbelievable tension at home as we struggled to hold our family, and our marriage, together under the strain.

So Lydia's issues weren't *caused* by tensions at home; they *were* the cause of the tension!

Therapists also overlooked the fact that Lydia was unable to express herself at school, either in the classroom or within her peer group. Fitting in is so very important for teenagers and I feel strongly that more help should be available for kids who find this difficult.

I began to be concerned about Lydia's eating - or, rather, the fact that she *wasn't* eating, on top of all the other trauma.

It was while we were on holiday in France that the alarm bells began to ring louder to the extent that I popped her onto the scales in a supermarket to see how much she weighed. I was shocked, so much so that I took her to see a paediatrician over there. It sounds crazy but I asked the paediatrician to check all my kids over at the same time so it wouldn't stress Lydia too much. I also asked him to *please tell Lydia to eat!*

So you can imagine my dismay when the paediatrician turned round and told us that his own daughter was much the same weight as Lydia and so, in his opinion, she was fine. He insisted that, with so many children being overweight these days, being slim was "a good thing". This, despite the fact that Lydia hadn't had a period for months.

Of course Lydia - or rather Lydia's emerging anorexia - latched onto this immediately. The paediatrician had said she was okay and so, to her increasingly malnourished mind, that meant she was. But deep down I am convinced that she was disappointed with his reaction. I believe that, inside, these children long to cry out for help but the eating disorder just won't let them.

By this time I'd begun to develop a great distrust of "experts". This was the reason why I hadn't taken Lydia to see the GP when I was worried she might be developing OCD (Obsessive Compulsive Disorder). And here we were with another professional who was claiming my daughter was absolutely fine when, clearly, she was not.

Anyway, back in the UK, I took Lydia to see our GP. She was a young doctor and very kind. I think she was quite inexperienced because she kept going off and checking Lydia's symptoms with more senior GPs. Well, by now I was pretty sure that we were dealing with anorexia. But the doctor said that it wasn't unusual for young girls to have irregular periods and asked us to come back in two weeks' time.

So we did.

In fact we went on to see a string of GPs and I couldn't believe what I was hearing. One even told Lydia that she needed to "get more of a life" and that, in her present state, she didn't stand a chance of getting into university, especially as she seemed to have virtually no interests.

It was as if Lydia had been sucked dry of all her personality and zest for life. But, to me, this had to be a symptom of the emerging anorexia.

Like any parent, I expect, I'd been scouring the internet for clues as to what was affecting my daughter. All the signs seemed to point to an eating disorder. But the GPs weren't convinced; they just kept telling us to come back in a few weeks' time to check how things were going.

By now I was frantic. To me it was as clear as day that Lydia had anorexia and I wanted them to act before it got worse. Instinctively I knew she had to eat so I wanted help in putting together a meal plan. But I'd no idea how to do this - or how to get her to eat once I'd done it!

We finally managed to get a GP to refer Lydia to CAMHS. Not for the eating disorder because, at this point it hadn't been officially diagnosed, but primarily because of her history of OCD and because she was behaving so strangely.

Curiously, no OCD was ever diagnosed. And it was a long time before we got a diagnosis of an eating disorder. Initially we went to see some people who, it appeared, were there to investigate whether or not she had an eating disorder. They asked Lydia: "What do you eat?" followed by: "You need to eat a bit more!" They advised her to eat lots of biscuits. We were given a questionnaire and it came back with "no eating disorder" as the diagnosis. We had to take her out from school for these sessions; it was GCSE year and the entire exercise would take a whole day, much of which was driving to and from the hospital.

Then the actual CAMHS appointment came through; we were to see them in two months' time. But, with an emerging eating disorder, a lot can happen in two months. Things went from bad to worse, and then even deeper as Lydia plummeted into the abyss. Often it seemed as if the only thing we ever did in our household was to yell at each other or spend hours at the dinner table with me pleading with Lydia to "just eat". Meanwhile she got thinner and thinner, and her moods and behaviours became more extreme.

Finally the day of the CAMHS appointment arrived and I thought, at last, we're going to get a proper diagnosis. So we sat there while Lydia completed another questionnaire. The consultant looked at it and - to my dismay - concluded that she wasn't suffering from an eating disorder. Also, the consultant completely ignored the OCD.

I was stunned! But more than anything, I was terrified. By this stage I knew that Lydia was hurtling into anorexia; it couldn't have been more obvious if it had hit me in the face... all those hours of pleading with her to eat... all that yelling... all those distressing behaviours that seemed to be getting more extreme by the day... not to mention the weight loss. Yet here were the professionals telling us - again - that she was perfectly okay!

In fact the consultant became quite accusative towards me. She was positively scary. She didn't speak; she shouted: "How do you have dinner?" or something along those lines, to which I'd reply "Well, we sit around the dinner table as a family, is this what you mean?"

It was as if they wanted to blame me. I was told in no uncertain terms that I must attend some carers' sessions. But, with all the driving, that would have eaten three or four hours out of my day and

I have a young son to look after, not to mention having to cope with everything that was going on with Lydia. I just couldn't make it. But the consultant barked at me that I didn't appear to understand how life-threatening this was.

Oh, believe me, I did understand. I most certainly did...

Then she'd bark at Lydia: "Why are you so shy?" And when Lydia didn't reply, she'd turn to me and bark: "Why is she so shy?"

"Er, well, because it's part of the problem," I'd respond, thinking that this was blatantly obvious.

It was dreadful, it really was.

Anyway by hook or by crook I managed to get Lydia to gain half a kilo by the next appointment. I told her how pleased I was with her, understanding that she would be frightened and needed encouragement.

But the consultant shouted at me that it wasn't enough. She put the fear of God into me - and into Lydia. As a result Lydia lost a whole kilo the following week - and she continued to lose weight. Her mood deteriorated and she began to isolate herself more than ever.

I took her back to the GP who weighed her and noted the weight loss. I insisted that she should be admitted to hospital, but was informed that no beds were available. And still Lydia hadn't been formally diagnosed with anorexia!

We were crawling up the wall with desperation by now. Our daughter was disappearing in front of our eyes yet no-one seemed the slightest bit interested!

I begged the consultant to have Lydia admitted. By this time Lydia was off school and the situation was becoming rapidly more painful. I would take her out to a coffee shop, for example, and she would take over an hour to finish her drink. Her OCD returned with a vengeance, so much so that on at least one occasion I remember her stopping suddenly in the middle of the shopping mall and - despite her shyness - performing a few minutes of ritual. Well, her weight went down and her problems got worse and worse... There was nothing I could do. I felt so very, very helpless. I saw no other way out than hospital admission.

But the scary consultant said there weren't any beds in our local NHS hospital. So, in desperation, I called a private hospital which charged an eye-watering £1,000 a day. Thankfully we had private medical insurance, a perk that came with my husband's job. The insurance company agreed to fund the admission.

So finally Lydia was admitted to the private hospital as a day patient. Gradually these became half days and then weekly appointments comprising a mixture of family therapy, individual therapy and sessions with a dietician.

Unfortunately things got a bit bumpy around the time of Lydia's GCSE examinations. She wasn't able to see the dietician regularly and, at other times, the dietician's diary was fully booked. Then came the summer holidays.

By the time September came along the dietician was shocked to see the change in Lydia and tried her best to make up for lost time. But it was a case of too little too late. By now Lydia's behaviour was impossible. She was getting increasingly violent towards me and hadn't gained any weight at all. But it took months for us to convince the dietician that Lydia wasn't just cutting back on food, she wasn't drinking either. She was severely dehydrated; the whites of her eyes were yellow. I also told the dietician about the little weights I'd discovered that Lydia had ordered online, presumably to trick the dietician into thinking she'd gained weight when she hadn't.

Thankfully all of this was enough to prompt the dietician into organising a hospital admission. It took a bit of organising, but two days later Lydia was admitted into the private hospital. But after a while, the insurance money ran out and so she went back to CAMHS (although we paid for her to stay with the private dietician because she was working wonders with our daughter).

After our experiences with the scary consultant, we were all nervous about what to expect with CAMHS. But we needn't have worried. The scary consultant had gone and we were put under the care of a new one, a lovely woman who actually listened to what we were saying. I can tell you it was such a relief to be finally listened to after all this time.

Anorexia is notorious for isolating its victims and, ever since she lost her confidence at primary school, Lydia had tended to keep herself isolated from her peers. When I suggested that Lydia and others might benefit from coaching on social skills, the consultant went away and set about organising a special social skills group. I felt this was good because they weren't just treating the symptoms, they were recognising that they needed to make functioning adults out of these young people.

The only trouble was that, before the group was launched, Lydia reached the age of 18 and no longer qualified for CAMHS. Now that she was legally permitted to make her own decisions about treatment, Lydia refused to move onto Adult Services. Legally, there was nothing I could do to make her go.

Right now, I am hoping to convince her to give Adult Services a try although, to be honest, I don't know much about them at all. To me, Adult Services seems quite a mysterious entity!

But it frustrates me so much that there is this cut-off point at 18 that totally disrupts everything and removes any continuity of care. It's almost as if, up until 18, there's all this support and then they're suddenly cut adrift. Or at least that's the way it seems to me.

For Lydia, it's been very disrupting. Because of her issues, she doesn't handle change well and she's finding this sudden move from a world where she feels safe to the daunting prospect of Adult Services quite frightening. This is the worst possible change that could have happened to her at this time.

The other problem is that, because with Lydia there is more going on than "just" an eating disorder, we need to find someone who is equipped to treat all of her issues or she'll come unstuck.

But the good news is that she is still seeing the private dietician every couple of weeks. The bad news is that she has been losing weight and is getting very depressed. Her OCD behaviours are also becoming more evident again. For example today she told me that she would increase her calories, but she'll only do things in multiples of three. For example, increasing her calories by 300, microwaving food for three minutes and so on. I strongly believe she needs some more therapy to help her deal with these issues as well as helping her to overcome the eating disorder behaviour, both of which appear to be related in our case.

These days Lydia's BMI is still very low. In fact it's within the anorexia diagnosis range and she lives off veg pots and porridge. But she is back at school and her social life has improved.

However, had her treatment been permitted to continue once she reached the "magic" age of 18, I believe we could have made real, positive progress. As it is, things aren't ideal and I can't help thinking that it needn't be this way; that it's crazy for the NHS to spend so much time and money on a patient only to cut them adrift once they reach 18.

What I wish more than anything is that Lydia could have continued treatment with CAMHS and that she could have attended that social skills group which, ironically, the psychiatrist had set up as a result of my suggestion.

With someone like Lydia who doesn't handle any type of change well, continuity of treatment is vital. But, as things currently stand, this isn't permitted to happen once they become an "adult".

Forget about the fact that, by this time, she was getting on with her new CAMHS treatment team like a house on fire and had built up a good relationship with them. They were achieving things that, back in those dreadful early days, we could never have dreamed possible. We really thought that, yes, this was it. With their amazing help, Lydia was going to recover. We were going to get our "little girl" back.

But then the ties were cut - snip! And we're having to start all over again. That is if I can convince her, as a legal adult who is permitted to make her own decisions, to say yes to further treatment.

Looking back, I think one of the hardest things was that, as her parent, I felt totally responsible for Lydia's recovery. If it had been cancer, for instance, I wouldn't have hesitated to trust the clinicians - and doubtless we would have received prompt and excellent treatment. They would have taken over the responsibility from me.

But with anorexia - or at least in my own personal experience of dealing with anorexia - it's as if no-one cares. The alarm bells just didn't go off - not with our GPs, not with CAMHS. And meanwhile my daughter was plummeting into this horrible illness. So it's down to the parents to constantly coach and support the child. But at the end of the day, we are just parents, we are not clinicians. We don't have formal training; all we have is what we've gleaned from books, the internet and talking with other families. And it's just so very, very draining. I remember being crushingly exhausted.

And when you're exhausted, you're not in the best place to deliver good care to your child. Meanwhile you've got your child's siblings to look after. You've got the school run, you've got meals to cook and, often, you've got a career to hold down. You are juggling a stack of balls at the same time and it's difficult to find the right balance. In a way, I've found it easier to accept the fact that, because of this, there are moments when you just can't help any more.

But, despite this, I will continue to fight for the best treatment for my child because that's what she still is: a child. Even though the law considers her to be an adult.

Yes, if I could wave a magic wand I'd get her back in front of that CAMHS treatment team, the team who was working so well with her after she left the private hospital. The team who, I believe, could have guided her towards a good all-round recovery regardless of whether she was 8, 18 or even 80.

Dawn's story

"These days Karen will spend time with friends and will eat what they are eating. They'll have a pizza, even go across the road to the chip shop and have a deep fried Mars Bar. Who would have thought it?"

Back at the start I never realised that it would take so long. When my daughter, Karen, was in the residential eating disorders clinic first time round I remember going along to one of the parents' meetings and thinking: "Oh, I'll only be here for a few weeks." I really thought you could fix this like you can a cold or an infection. Then, several years down the line, you realise that there is no quick fix; it's a long old haul. But, thankfully, our story has a happy ending, and the last eight months or so have been entirely down to Karen's sheer grit and determination to recover.

As a girl, Karen was always lively, chatty and outgoing with lots of friends. She was also a bit of a perfectionist. Even at primary school she'd insist that everything she wrote in her school exercise books had to be nice and neat, and if it wasn't then she'd rub it all out and start again.

But Karen had always enjoyed food; in fact she loved to try all kinds of different foods. She would eat anything we put in front of her.

I think she was probably about 13 or 14 when I first began to notice something. One day she came to me and said she wanted to go and see a doctor because she was having "funny thoughts". The GP diagnosed her with OCD and she was referred to CAMHS. But she was referred as an OCD patient rather than an eating disorder patient. At the time she was still eating fine.

Then, when she was probably about 14, she began to get more obsessive about what size clothes she was wearing. She also became a bit fussier about food - all the usual excuses like, "I've eaten at school" or "I'm not hungry, I'm eating later on with my friends".

I'd also begun to find bits of paper hidden around the house with lists of what she'd eaten and how many calories she'd had. She'd totalled it up to around 600 or 700 calories a day, but in reality it was more like 300 calories. Karen started to have things like half a kiwi for breakfast, claiming that she couldn't eat any more because she felt sick, she'd have more at lunchtime or she'd eat on the way to school. I mentioned the calorie lists to her CAMHS therapist and asked if she could probe this a little bit more.

The therapist came back saying that she'd spoken to Karen but Karen had assured her that she was eating properly, that she wasn't trying to lose any weight and that it was just normal teenage behaviour.

I wasn't convinced.

I brought it up again because I was noticing even more calorie lists. I pointed out that Karen was losing weight, that she wasn't eating properly and that it wasn't just a normal teenage thing.

Thankfully they took me seriously and we began to see a fantastic eating disorders therapist called Susan. She cottoned on straight away and realised exactly what Karen was doing. But Karen began to get angry about the fact that her cover had been blown and she refused to go to the next appointment.

One day Susan called me at work to say: "You need to get Karen to a GP now, today, and get her referred to the hospital because we need to do a full check."

Our usual GP was off work and I was put onto another doctor. I explained that I needed an urgent appointment and why - exactly what Susan had told me to say. But he just brushed it off saying: "I don't see the urgency. I can't just refer you. Call me back in a week if she isn't any better."

So I phoned Susan right back and told her. She was furious and told me to phone back again and demand an appointment. She said she'd give me her direct phone number and I was to tell the doctor to phone her. So I called the surgery again. This time I spoke to a lovely doctor who gave us a double appointment and rang Susan who explained the urgency. This doctor got us an appointment at the hospital for the very next day.

We spent eight hours or so in the paediatric ward as the medical staff checked Karen over before arranging for her to go to a private residential eating disorders clinic the following day. Her treatment was to be funded by the NHS. By this time Karen's weight was extremely low. I can still see her, lying on that bed while the doctors were doing all that prodding and blood pressure checking. I was shocked. I couldn't believe how tiny and ill she looked. You see, I hadn't seen her without any clothes on for ages because, whenever I saw her, she'd always be in baggy tee-shirts, sweaters and jogging bottoms.

So we went along to the private clinic.

But getting to this stage hadn't been easy. First I'd had to convince CAMHS to take the calorie counting seriously. Then I'd had to get past that first GP and eventually get a referral to the hospital. I dread to think what the outcome might have been if we hadn't had someone as formidable as Susan on the team. She was great. Mind you, Karen hated her with a passion. Susan was very, very strict and you couldn't pull the wool over her eyes. She didn't care whether you liked her or not. She said she wasn't there to be liked; she was there to get Karen well. She was absolutely fantastic.

Karen was at the private clinic for about six months. They were very good. Karen kind of played along. She was the model patient and did everything she was supposed to do, but basically this was just so she could get out of the place. Once discharged, it didn't take her very long to go back downhill again.

Next, Karen was referred to a specialist eating disorders service.

We saw them once a week. By this time she was very weak and underweight. She was managing to squirrel away food; I was finding discarded food for ages afterwards in all kinds of strange and bizarre places. In the end Karen was referred back to our local hospital where she stayed for around ten days on complete bed rest.

I took all her food into the paediatric ward and stayed with her while she was there. I gave her special build-up drinks which she somehow managed to avoid drinking. The tricks she used in order to avoid eating and drinking were nothing less than ingenious. She also managed to trick the staff into thinking she weighed more than she actually did. In fact the sheer lengths she'd go to deceive everyone were horrifying.

Anyway, Karen was discharged back to the eating disorders service. But, by now, she was just getting rid of everything I was giving her. I'd find discarded or regurgitated food stashed everywhere. I'd taken six months off work so I could be at home with her because she wasn't able to go to school. But she was still managing to lose weight. Eventually, at one of her appointments, she refused to be weighed. And nothing they said or did would persuade her otherwise; it didn't matter whether they were nice or strict, she just wasn't responding. In the event they did manage to weigh her and insisted that, at this weight, she needed to be referred back to the private clinic urgently. This was March 2010.

When she was weighed at the private clinic her weight was actually much, much lower - alarmingly almost twenty-five-per-cent lower. She had obviously managed to fool the eating disorders service into thinking she weighed more than she did. And they'd thought she was really sick at the fake weight!

Karen was in the private clinic for about eighteen months. This time round she fought the treatment much more; she was no longer the model patient. She hated eating and she hated having to put on weight. So she just resurrected all the food hiding tricks she'd been using at home. Patients were watched very well, round the clock, yet somehow she still managed to fool them, often in even more shocking and ingenious ways.

On top of this she was self-harming, often quite dangerously, like the day she locked herself in the hospital cleaning cupboard where all the cleaning fluids were stored. That resulted in a quick rush to the local general hospital which scared the life out of me.

The hospital told Karen that they wouldn't discharge her until she had something to eat. Of course, to Karen, this gave her the green light *not* to eat, but they didn't seem to understand this. At the private clinic every missed calorie would be replaced with a build-up drink or nasogastric tube, so naturally I wanted her back there as soon as possible to avoid any more weight loss. So I pushed for a discharge, emphasising the fact that we'd bring her back to the hospital if there were any complications once she began to take in food. I still find it frustrating that the general hospital appeared to know so little about the ins and outs of eating disorders.

During those eighteen months at the private clinic I think something began to shift inside her head. Karen gradually began to realise that she didn't want that kind of life anymore, but she was struggling to find a way back to normality. When she was discharged, I managed to get a referral back to the eating disorders service. I was surprised that this wasn't set up automatically, but for some reason it wasn't.

Karen was given a lovely therapist who helped her enormously - not necessarily with the food but with thinking about her life in general. She got her to aim for certain goals that weren't necessarily based around food. They were based around going to college and what she was going to study at college or do in the future, about going out with her friends and so on.

We did have a couple of strange appointments with the consultant psychiatrist who said things like: "Well if you're not going to do this or that, then do you want me to discharge you?" And, yes, I think she would have discharged her. In the end Karen *was* discharged and she was still underweight.

Curiously, however, things began to get better after we left the service, maybe because she no longer had somebody telling her what to do all the time.

From then on it was just the two of us fighting for her recovery. Well, to be truthful, it was mostly Karen who did all the fighting. She was pretty awesome, really.

Eight or nine months on she still struggles and she'll still ask me if it's okay to eat something, for instance can she have some cheese and crackers, or can she go and get some chocolate. But she eats everything, which is great news, and her weight is back to normal.

These days she'll spend time with friends and will eat what they are eating. They'll come round here and they'll sit and have a pizza, even go across the road to the chip shop and have a deep fried Mars Bar. Who would have thought it? I think that being with her friends and having a normal life is one of the things that spurred her on.

But I would definitely say that Karen has done most of the hard work herself. Also by being brave enough to go back to college, to see people, make new friends and to move on.

There is still a little way to go. But Karen, being the strong and determined person she is, will get there. I am certain of it.

Heather's story

"While our child is being treated, we are busy learning too. And, unlike the professionals, we have no-one coaching us. All we have are books, internet sources and anyone else we can find whose brains are willing to be picked."

There's a poem about a little girl that goes: "When she was good she was very, very good - but when she was bad she was horrid." This pretty much sums up my daughter Ruth who, as a toddler, would have violent tantrums two or three times a day when she would bang her head against things and scream for long periods. Yet at other times she could be an absolute delight.

Ruth was always bright and academically way ahead of her peers at school although, socially, she was very immature. For her there was no middle ground; it was one extreme or another. As a result her teachers either adored her or found her impossible.

Since birth, Ruth had suffered from low blood sugar. When the blood sugar dropped, her tantrums would kick off and so we were always careful to ensure she ate regular meals. Ruth also had problems sleeping. She'd had problems feeding as a baby, but once she reached toddlerhood she seemed relatively okay although she refused to take anything that wasn't very sweet from a spoon.

Ruth was nine when my husband, David, suffered his first bout of depression. At the time I was struggling with a fulfilling but very demanding job and, of course, there was our younger daughter, Amy, to think about as well. So my attention was deflected away from

Ruth's emerging problems for a year or so.

When she was eleven, Ruth won a place at a highly academic secondary school on the other side of town. She found it hard to settle and had a lot of meltdowns during that first year. It took Ruth and the school some time to get used to each other!

She struggled with the gap between early breakfast and late lunch, and started snacking in between meals on chocolate from the school vending machines. She began to put on weight and was teased by some of the boys. So I was actually relieved when, aged 13, she began to lose weight and settle in a bit more at school.

Meanwhile David's depression came back. At the time I was working even longer hours and Amy was busy changing schools. So, again, I put my worries about Ruth onto a backburner. As a result I failed to notice that she was beginning to develop an eating disorder.

A couple of other incidents happened around this time which may have triggered the descent. The first was to do with her small but intense group of friends. Some of them had been "experimenting" with cutting and overdosing - and one girl in particular had begun to exhibit some really disturbing behaviour.

The second was that Ruth fell in love. When the boy ended the relationship Ruth threw herself into an almost melodramatic steep decline. She'd spend hours crying up in her room. She began to cut and burn her legs, and on one occasion she took a small overdose. She was also cutting back on her food. It didn't help that, as a Christian family, we were being quite strict for Lent. But when Easter came and the rest of the family indulged in Easter eggs and cake, Ruth didn't. She either made excuses to skip meals or she over-ate, punishing herself with cuts and crying fits afterwards.

Worried, I went to see our GP who insisted it was probably a "phase" and that I shouldn't worry too much. But of course I did worry. Then one day, frightened by a particularly out of control binge, Ruth took herself off to the see the GP. The doctor immediately diagnosed anorexia, sent off a referral and promptly left on a six month sabbatical.

During the two months we waited for the appointment to come through, David and I read up on eating disorders. However the information seemed to be conflicting. On one hand the books were telling us that we shouldn't make an issue about food and we should trust the professionals to get our child well. On the other hand they said that, as our child was under 16, we might be expected to re-feed her as a family and that the professionals would teach us how to do this. So we weren't sure what to expect.

The whole family turned up as instructed for the first specialist appointment: Ruth, David, Amy and me. We saw two clinicians while another two observed from behind a two-way mirror.

During a very difficult 40 minutes they asked us all kinds of questions which extended to the problems we'd had over David's depression and also the fact that a (adopted) cousin of mine had died from anorexia. I remember my younger daughter, Amy, just sitting there in bewildered silence, overwhelmed by the whole thing.

They suggested we get hold of a book - *A Parents' Guide to Eating Disorders* - which we bought and read avidly, and that was really that. We staggered out of the appointment really none the wiser.

The book argued that parents needed to take control of their child's eating. The only problem was that it failed to say *how* we were supposed to do this. Parental unity, it insisted, was key. Parents would act together as a team to work out the best way to help their child. No professional guidance would be given on how to do this as the parents would know the child best. So, armed with this (quite scary) information, we went along to a second session with the professionals.

We were seen by two people: a social worker called Alan and a young woman called Lucy who was to be Ruth's individual therapist. Initially I didn't have much confidence in either of them and it didn't help that the appointment was on 9/11, the same day as the Twin Towers attacks. We emerged from the session into a changed world. All we did when we got home was to telephone all our relatives in New York to check they were okay.

As the world gradually recovered from the initial shock of 9/11, I attempted to get Ruth to eat. She agreed to have breakfast and, in a bid to help curb her bingeing, she asked me to stop stocking snack foods. But she wasn't eating school dinners. As a result she lost more weight.

Alan urged us to make her eat more but failed to tell us how to do it. I left the next session angry and confused. Ruth became distressed at the clinic and, as soon as we got home, she ran away. My husband took to his bed, Amy took off to a friend's house and I took to the streets to look for Ruth, eventually finding her lying in the road in the dark threatening to kill herself.

Desperate to find a way of getting Ruth to eat and put on weight, I had a word with a doctor friend of mine - Mary - to see if she could help out with some dietetic support and devise a weight-gain eating plan. Her advice was excellent. However Ruth was unable to stick to the plan properly. Her weight flat-lined, but at least she wasn't losing.

Well, Alan was furious with me! How dare I bring in a third party without his knowledge! But the psychiatrist didn't seem to have a problem with it. So we were getting mixed messages.

Meanwhile things seemed to be going a little better on the eating front. Ruth was managing four "meals" a day including a large build-up drink with the evening meal. I went into school to supervise her lunches and I'm pleased to say that the school was dealing quite well with her outbursts. Mary's scales showed that she was slowly gaining weight and the suicide threats and cutting abated a little.

But far from working together as a "team", my husband David and I were having our own issues. David was becoming increasingly angry and depressed at Ruth's behaviour and tried to avoid spending time in the house. So it was all a bit one-sided and there was a great deal of tension.

We brought up the subject at the next family session. Alan's reaction was that it wasn't surprising that things were getting tricky; we shouldn't have followed Mary's advice, we should have simply got our daughter to eat. He insisted that, until we got her to eat and she put on weight, there wouldn't be any progress. But just how were we supposed to get our daughter to eat? She wouldn't eat for us. She *couldn't* eat for us. Yet here we were being condemned for failing to do something that we hadn't been taught how to do. We also felt we were being condemned for bringing in Mary to help. We felt as if we were on our own, killing our child through our own stupidity. We felt terrible.

If Ruth wouldn't eat at home, Alan said, then she would have to be admitted to hospital. Ruth jumped at the idea. "Yes please," she said, she would love to go to hospital. Again, we left in confusion and despair. And again, Ruth ran out of the house as soon as we got home. I wrote a curt letter to Alan along the lines of "If you think it's so easy then YOU feed her!"

I took Ruth back to the GP - a new GP, Dr Harrison, who proved to be a lot more successful, in my opinion, than the eating disorders team. To be truthful I think Dr Harrison saved my marriage, my sanity and quite possibly my daughter's life.

Dr Harrison was one of those people that adored Ruth and it was mutual. She told Ruth in no uncertain terms that she needed to eat more, but she recognised how difficult it was to get someone with anorexia to eat. She herself had had a roommate at medical school who had suffered from anorexia so she'd seen it for herself.

Unlike the Eating Disorders Team, she treated Ruth like an adult and Ruth appreciated this. If nothing else, her insight and sense of humour managed to keep Ruth safe, even if it didn't "cure" her of her anorexia.

Back at therapy we found ourselves in front of the Team Leader: Martin. He wanted us to be firm but appeared to be receptive to our problems. Also, he wasn't keen on having Ruth admitted to a unit; it would be a last resort. Meanwhile David hoped that, as the Team Leader, Martin would be able to fix things. On Martin's instructions I continued to push the eating while Ruth continued to have meltdowns and David got angry, spending more and more time out of the house.

Then Ruth took her second overdose. In her suicide note she blamed me, stating that "Ana" (anorexia) was all she wanted to live for. She was admitted to the children's ward in our local hospital where the staff interviewed her, identified problems with schoolwork as a contributing factor and discharged her.

Back home I continued to insist that Ruth ate. She was furious with me and promptly admitted herself back to hospital. There she was assessed by Martin and a new psychiatrist who seemed more interested in our marital problems than the matter of getting Ruth to eat and get well. David wanted Ruth to be admitted to the eating disorders unit and when Martin refused, he stormed out of the building in anger.

I took Ruth back home. On Martin's instructions I pressed less but still tried to be firm with the food. The idea was that we were to draw the focus away from the eating and concentrate more on communication issues within the family. Well of course this just got David's back up. He became even more hostile to the team and even more angry with Ruth and myself.

I now realise that he was acting entirely out of fear, but at the time it was as if he hated us. David wanted Ruth hospitalised, or medicated, or both, and above all cured. He just wanted something *to be done* rather than all this faffing about.

Increasingly, I found myself using the therapy appointments to express my anger at David. Martin suggested marital therapy. David didn't want to play ball. He refused to go to sessions. In the end the "family sessions" comprised solely of Ruth and me sitting in front of Martin and sometimes - bless her - Dr Harrison.

We continued to muddle through and Ruth's weight remained stable. She still spoke of suicide but at least she was no longer running in front of cars or taking overdoses. However David's mood didn't improve. Amy spent a lot of time away from the home and her schoolwork suffered. I was eventually advised to back off totally from the eating and Ruth relaxed a bit. She gained a bit of weight and, almost two years after our first appointment, had a period and was discharged from treatment.

Of course she wasn't "cured", but at least she was safe and being monitored by Dr Harrison. I did toy with the idea of getting back in touch with the specialists but the sessions had been so awful and had caused so much upset within the home that I thought better of it.

By this time I had made contact with other parents in the world of eating disorders. Their advice was mixed. Many advised "backing off" and avoiding "enmeshment" while others used expensive "residential" therapy or insisted on NHS inpatient treatment.

Then I met Laura Collins.

As the Founder of the charity F.E.A.S.T. and author of the book *Eating With Your Anorexic*, Laura was different.

She was a powerful advocate for Family-Based Treatment (FBT), often known as the Maudsley Approach, where you focus on re-feeding your child first and deal with the cognitive issues later. Behind the scenes, Laura - who lives in the States - became a good friend and helped me to understand the models Alan and Martin had tried to use. The only problem was that, try as I might, I'd been unable to put FBT into practice as far as our own situation was concerned.

I felt an enormous sense of guilt about this.

Meanwhile our family plodded on. Ruth was neither dying nor cured. If you saw her back then you'd think her pretty if a bit slight in build. But looks can be deceptive. Underneath the lovely appearance, her periods had stopped again. On the other hand she was just about coping with school, had passed her examinations and had established a small group of good friends.

Her moods went up and down. But this wasn't unusual; Ruth had always been like this.

So, really, it was like this: Ruth was still sick, but she wasn't sick enough to get (or want) treatment. And, anyway, the treatment she had received had almost ended our marriage and there simply weren't any other local treatment teams available.

When Ruth reached 18 she started at a local college. By not

choosing the more stressful university option, I hoped that things would get easier for her and that she would thrive. Meanwhile Dr Harrison left the area. Now Ruth and I were on our own: no familiar teachers, no familiar doctor. Both of us felt quite lost. And all the local eating disorders team could offer was a course of CBT. But because Ruth was now classed as an adult she had to "want" to have it. She turned down the offer; it sounded too much like hard work.

She desperately tried to fit in at college and she worked hard, got good grades and impressed the tutors. She also got herself a part-time job and was desperately trying to build up her social circle. Meanwhile she was eating very little. So I dragged a very thin Ruth along to see Alan at his new office. He was horrified at the sight of her and incredibly gentle and sensible. But, because she was an adult and none of us knew what she weighed (and she wasn't giving anyone permission to weigh her), legally we could do nothing.

We discussed getting her sectioned under the Mental Health Act to "force" her to have treatment. Thankfully in the end Ruth agreed to be weighed. We were all horrified to discover that her BMI had dropped to just 12. It terrified Ruth. So much so that she attempted to eat her way out of it. Over the next two weeks (which happened to be Christmas) bingeing, interspersed with panic overdoses, made her both physically and mentally unstable.

Thankfully, after Christmas, Ruth agreed to Alan's offer of an emergency placement in the adult specialist unit. Things weren't easy there, but the staff were kind and Ruth's weight was restored.

Post discharge, we have had our ups and downs and I certainly can't say that Ruth is fully cured, but she has maintained a healthy enough weight for several years now.

Me, well, I carry an awful lot of guilt. I often wonder what would have happened if I'd listened more closely to David and insisted on getting Ruth admitted sooner rather than later. Would she be well today? Did I, by following what I felt was the right route at the time, inadvertently prolong my daughter's illness or make it worse?

The fact is that, as parents, we embark on this journey knowing very little. While our child is undergoing treatment, we are busy learning too. And, unlike the professionals, we have no-one coaching us. All we have are books, internet sources and anyone else we can find along the way whose brains are willing to be picked.

So I keep telling myself that I mustn't feel guilty. It is not anyone's fault that Ruth's treatment was so haphazard and slow. Also, Ruth had always had problems, ever since the day she was born. She had had various other psychiatric diagnoses over the years and, while none of them have yet "stuck", the majority of clinicians who have known her are convinced that her problem was not "just" an eating disorder.

Nevertheless it doesn't stop me from feeling guilty. But we're all still alive. We're all still together. Ruth has a lovely boyfriend who wants her to be well enough to live with him as an equal and not as an invalid. She is also a proud aunt, Amy having grown up lively and strong and started a family of her own.

MY TIP:

Don't be afraid to question the professionals. If something is confusing you or just doesn't seem right, then say so. The professionals can't understand what is going on in your own home if you don't explain it, and sometimes it can take a lot of explaining!

Adrienne's story

"I needed someone to hold my hand and tell me how to help my daughter but no-one seemed to have any answers. I felt totally helpless, isolated and very frightened. It was overwhelming."

Even though it's only been six months since Lucy's diagnosis, I still find it difficult to recall my feelings and attitudes towards anorexia prior to this. I had read the usual sensationalist stories in newspapers and magazines. I had seen photos of severely emaciated young girls and I remember the tragic Karen Carpenter story from years ago.

I expect that, like many people, I thought of anorexia as an illness of the rich and famous - or girls who had serious childhood issues. I never thought that it could, and indeed does, happen to ordinary families and to boys as well as girls.

As a family, we were certainly not dysfunctional in any shape or form. In fact I'm sure that most people thought we "had it all". We were a typical traditional happy family. Lucy is the youngest of three children. She was by far the liveliest; I think she had to be lively to be heard over the other two! Back then I wouldn't have described her as a particularly anxious child, nor do I remember her being a perfectionist. Also, she was quite shy amongst people she didn't know. She was never one to join clubs outside school or to stay away from home for too long. Now, with hindsight, she possibly did suffer from a mild form of social and separation anxiety, but nothing unusual. She really enjoyed school, was very popular amongst her peers and, as far as I'm aware, she had a very happy and secure childhood. We were very fortunate to be bringing up our family in such circumstances and we appreciated this and made sure our children didn't take it for granted.

Lucy's periods started when she was 13 and took us by surprise. She had always had a very slim athletic body, and still looked very much a child without a hint of puppy fat. Her older sister had a similar build and was nearly 16 when her periods started, so we assumed Lucy would begin at a similar age. Over the coming months Lucy seemed to grow and develop at an incredibly fast rate. This was frequently commented on by friends and family with statements such as "Gosh Lucy, you've grown" or "I hardly recognised her". Pretty typical things to say to teenagers, I expect.

Initially Lucy still seemed perfectly happy and adjusted. She wasn't at all moody and I thought we'd got off lightly with the whole teenage thing. Around three months later, in the summer of 2011, we went on holiday with my sister's family. I don't remember Lucy being particularly body-conscious and she seemed to enjoy playing in the pool with the others. She has since told me that she can remember disliking the way she looked on that holiday. I also noticed a bit of "attitude" creeping in, but nothing that we didn't put down to "teenage behaviour".

With hindsight I think this is the point when I believe Lucy's problems started to develop. When I look back at photographs of her with her friends, she had grown a lot taller and thinner than her peers. She was underweight. But I just didn't see it at the time.

September came and, with it, the start of a new term. Some days Lucy went without lunch at school. When I questioned her she would claim that the queues were "too long" or, since the school lunch hour had been cut to half an hour, she'd say she "didn't have time". In reality she was finding it increasingly difficult to eat in front of people. But, again, it didn't register in my mind that anything was wrong.

The "attitude" became worse over the next few months. Lucy wasn't argumentative as such; in fact she didn't seem to like talking to us or her siblings at all. Instead, she spent an awful lot of time on her computer or in her room. I'd describe her mood as "sullen".

She still had the same group of friends, plus a boyfriend. She still socialised well and her school reports continued to be good. We thought it was just typical teenage behaviour and that it would pass. The idea that Lucy could be developing an eating disorder never entered our heads.

Then, early in 2012, she started to have panic attacks. There seemed to be no reason for them. She'd panic that she would oversleep and be late for school. Or she'd just panic about having a panic attack. Having suffered from panic attacks myself in the past, I know it's a vicious circle and the more importance you place on them the worse they seem to get. I told her not to worry, to try and stay calm and they would pass.

Lucy also began to develop mysterious aches and pains. We visited the doctor several times but nothing was ever found. Meanwhile the panic attacks continued. But, to be honest, I didn't think this anxiety was really anything to worry about. Again, I just put it down to normal teenage angst.

Around this time Lucy also started to get overly concerned about school work and her impending GCSEs. Her brother and sister had both done well in their exams and I expect she felt pressure to do the same. But she couldn't decide on which GCSE options to choose or what career path she wanted to eventually take.

Lucy was also becoming very image conscious, constantly worrying about what other people were thinking of her. She seemed to need constant approval on what to wear, what to do or how to behave. Acceptance within her peer group became everything and her self-esteem appeared to have reached rock bottom. To me, my once carefree daughter had become an anxious and withdrawn teenager. She would spend hours on the computer, particularly social networking sites, checking her wall to see how many "likes" she had compared to others, rarely posting statuses for fear of ridicule and generally feeling unpopular. Meanwhile she was becoming a perfectionist, both in her schoolwork and appearance. She'd spend hours getting ready, doing her hair and makeup, never satisfied and always saying she looked awful or a "mess". Her school work would be done and then redone. Art homework would be crumpled up and thrown away as it wasn't "good enough". It seemed that nothing could ever be "good enough". She was never satisfied. But, if she became interested in something, then she would pursue it in an almost obsessional way.

Suddenly and without warning her boyfriend ended their relationship. They were so young and it had never gone beyond the "holding hands" stage, but he was a popular boy and the fact that she was his girlfriend gave her status. The very thing that had been keeping her afloat was gone. She felt rejected, unloved and unpopular. She cried all that evening and night but, strangely, the next day she claimed everything was fine and that she was "over" him. I think she bottled up her feelings; they were too painful to deal with. She tried to find another way to be liked.

Within weeks, unbeknown to me, she started to diet, dramatically cutting her calories to very low levels and visiting "pro-ana" websites, looking at pictures and getting tips on how to combat hunger and how to fool others into thinking she was eating.

But, of course, I had no idea that this was going on.

Then the exercising began. When her dad and I were out of the house, she'd use a video exercise game to monitor her weight loss and she began to exercise compulsively. If we ever questioned her about it, she'd insist that she was trying to get fit.

Often she claimed she wasn't able to finish her evening meal because she'd already eaten something when she came in from school. But, unbeknown to me, she hadn't had any breakfast or lunch. Meanwhile I was working longer hours, so I wasn't getting home until late. I'd arrive home to find debris in the kitchen left, I assumed, by my two daughters making things to eat earlier. And, because Lucy's lunch account was still being used, I assumed she was having the usual school lunches. Now I know these were either being thrown away or given to friends.

But still we noticed nothing.

In fact none of us picked up that anything was wrong, apart from Lucy's brother who, on his return from a gap year abroad, kept saying how ill she looked and how she had dark circles under her eyes probably, he claimed, as a result of spending too long in front of a computer. Because we saw her every day we hadn't noticed and, in any case, I assumed he was saying these things to wind her up.

Lucy did stop using the computer as much and instead filled her time with exercise. She was constantly drinking pints of water. I now know this was to "fill" her up. Despite her very slim appearance, Lucy had always been a "chocoholic" and loved takeaways, sweets, crisps, biscuits and so on. In the past we'd have terrible problems getting her to eat vegetables or salad. We'd be constantly pointing out how unhealthy her diet was becoming and that she should cut back on all the "junk food" she was having in-between meals.

So, when she began to ask if we could have salad more often and carried on exercising, I saw it as a positive sign that she wanted to live a more healthy and active lifestyle. I was actually pleased she was looking after herself.

Cleverly, she made sure she ate when we were all together. So, again, we didn't notice anything. But of course we were only together for that one meal a day. I had no idea that she was making up for it the following day or whenever she got a chance.

During the summer of 2012 Lucy went on holiday with a friend's family. I clicked onto a social networking site where her friend had posted some photos. I thought there was real sadness in Lucy's eyes. Yes, she was smiling, but it just didn't look genuine and I couldn't put my finger on it. I simply assumed she must be homesick.

Shortly afterwards we went on holiday as a family. To all intents and purposes, Lucy was eating normally. In fact she seemed perfectly normal. Even though she'd grown taller and was slim, she didn't look worryingly thin. But, once back home, she felt she needed to cut back to make up for everything she'd eaten while away. She whittled her intake down to just 250 - 500 calories a day. But we simply didn't notice.

Over the following weeks we had quite a few family celebrations. Lots of other things were going on during this period, too. We were having an extension built, we were busy getting the girls ready for school in September and we were frantically catching up on our work after the holidays. Lucy's restricting continued to go unnoticed.

I remember she kept asking how long dinner would be. She'd want to know what we were having and did she have to have this or that. She'd get very anxious whilst I was preparing the meal and would keep coming into the kitchen to check on progress. I was getting in from work later and later, so it could be quite late in the evening by the time we sat down for dinner. Looking back, she must have been absolutely starving, waiting for her only meagre meal of the day. But, even then, some of it would inevitably end up "accidentally" dropped on the floor, given to the dog, hidden or left because she didn't like it or had "eaten too much earlier".

I remember Lucy being so very cold all the time. She was always sitting on the Aga or in her room with the hairdryer on her trying to keep warm. She'd wear layers of baggy clothes and jumpers. It was a cold summer but, even with the extra clothes, she could never get warm. Her mood was very low, too. I remember her voice becoming barely audible, so much so that I could scarcely hear her at times. I thought my hearing was going!

I remember thinking how I wished she would hurry up and grow out of this horrible teenage stage. But I consoled myself with the thought that in a few months' time she'd be back to her old self.

In truth I stayed out of her way as much as possible to avoid conflict. If we were alone in the car, the journey would be spent in stony silence, or my questions would be answered with one-word replies. The atmosphere around her was awful and, if I am totally honest, my tolerance levels were getting low. But my other children had all had periods of moodiness as teenagers and I didn't think this was any different. I just assumed that, if I was patient, it would pass.

So I ignored it.

Lucy returned to school at the beginning of September 2012 but, increasingly, her friends seemed to irritate her. She'd come home saying she was "fed up with everyone", how she hated the people in her class and that they were getting on her nerves. She even asked if she could change schools so she could start afresh elsewhere.

This is when I started to suspect that something was wrong. But my focus was on school. Was she being bullied? Was she finding the work too hard? Wasn't she getting on with the teachers? Was the pressure of GCSEs too much?

The next morning was a Saturday. Lucy had a swimming lesson at 6am and we had to be up at 5am. By this time she must have been so weak that I've no idea how she managed it. On the way home, assuming she must be hungry, I bought her an iced doughnut - her favourite - to cheer her up. She didn't touch it. It stayed on her lap all the way home. I kept asking her what was wrong. Lucy said nothing and stared out of the window. She seemed angry and irritated by my questioning. I sat next to her, crying silently all the way home. She was emotionless, just a shell. I could have told her the dog had died and there would have been no response, nothing. It was awful and, by this stage, I was getting very worried.

I asked her repeatedly whether we'd done something to upset her. Was there anything we could help her with? But she wouldn't answer. So I told her I'd be taking her to the doctor on Monday. I was beginning to get frightened. I sensed that something was seriously wrong and that this wasn't "just teenage angst", but still I wasn't able to put the puzzle pieces together. I had no idea what I was looking at.

When we got home Lucy went to her room. I sat on the stairs outside listening to her sobbing. I was the one panicking now. What on earth could be wrong? My mind was frantically racing from one awful scenario to the next. In all honesty things were so bad I even wondered if she might have a brain tumour! Moments later she emerged red eyed and handed me a letter, saying: "You'd better read this."

The letter said that, for months, she'd been unhappy about her weight, so she'd been dieting and exercising. But now she was frightened as she didn't get hungry anymore. She felt cold, lethargic, dizzy and drowsy all the time and she was too scared to eat. She wasn't sure if she had an eating disorder. The realisation almost felt like the force of a physical explosion - BANG! - I knew instantly that she had an eating disorder. I went into her room, threw my arms around her and cried and cried.

Instinctively all weekend I tried to get food into her. As her mother that was my natural reaction. Meanwhile I was thinking: how on earth could this have happened without me noticing? All the strange behaviour around food, all the excuses, all the exercising, all the unhappiness... Finally it all made sense. I put the pieces of the puzzle together. Lucy had anorexia. I was in a state of blind panic.

There was so much emotion that weekend: the shock of discovery, the realisation of what we were dealing with and the guilt. There was so much guilt that I'd failed to cotton onto the fact my daughter had been literally starving herself for months. Why hadn't I picked up on all the signals? Why couldn't she have come to me when she was so desperately unhappy? Why had my very slim daughter thought she needed to lose weight? I am still plagued by these thoughts today.

That weekend I fed her all her favourites; whatever I could think of just to get some food inside her. She refused; she cried and said she couldn't eat. It was horrific and unbearable to watch. It was just unthinkable that this could be happening to my daughter. And the more she confessed to what had been going on the worse I felt.

Unbelievably on the Monday morning Lucy went to school. Meanwhile I made two emergency appointments with the doctor: one for me and one for both of us together.

The GP was truly amazing; she was so understanding. She had children the same age and she'd known Lucy since she was a baby. After Lucy had left the room we shed a few tears together. The GP obviously knew the battle that was ahead of us. She admitted that her knowledge of eating disorders was limited but, despite this, I am so, so grateful to her for recognising the seriousness of the situation, for not dismissing my concerns and for acting so promptly. She weighed Lucy and explained that, as Lucy's weight was so low, she would arrange an emergency appointment with the local CAMHS team but that it might be several weeks before we were seen. She also did blood tests, and checked her heart and blood pressure. Both were very low, indeed her blood sugar was at a dangerous level. The GP monitored her very closely over the next few days and weeks, and I made sure she was eating at home, although this was getting increasingly difficult.

That first weekend Lucy had been reasonably compliant. Yes, she cried and begged me not to give her food and make her "fat", but although it was hard for her, she did eat.

Gradually over the coming weeks, however, that initial compliance disappeared. It surprised me how quickly things became much, much worse. She was adamant that there was nothing wrong with her; she was in complete denial. Her thinking was totally illogical; I couldn't make her see sense. In fact, the more explaining and reasoning we tried, the more determined she became. It was bewildering for all of us. The anorexia seemed to be tightening its grip and the real fight began. Mealtimes quickly became a battlefield; usually ending in angry outbursts of shouting or tears - or, more often, both. She'd get angry and violent. Sometimes she wouldn't allow us near her whereas other times she'd cry uncontrollably. It was heart-breaking.

It wasn't just the fact that getting food into her took so long; it was the fact that, after she'd eaten, she had to be consoled and distracted from her thoughts. She was often hysterical and it took every ounce of energy to calm her down. We began to realise the enormity of what we were dealing with and it was unbearable. Frequently each meal ran into the next. Our whole family life was turned upside down. In fact it's not an exaggeration to say that it was as if some evil entity had "possessed" Lucy. She was unrecognisable.

I tried to find help but I didn't know who to turn to. Every book or article I read seemed to have different, usually conflicting, views. It was all so confusing. I needed someone to hold my hand and tell me how to help my daughter but no-one seemed to have any answers. I felt totally helpless, isolated and very frightened. It was overwhelming.

It seemed like an eternity but, in reality, it took three weeks for the CAMHS appointment to come through. I remember sitting in the waiting room trying to get my head around the fact that my daughter had a serious mental health problem when, weeks earlier, she had been sitting happily on the beach, laughing and messing around, seemingly without a care in the world. It just didn't make any sense at all.

I had so many questions, but my priority was Lucy. I would do anything to make her better. The first CAMHS session lasted two-and-a-half hours. Lucy was weighed, but despite my efforts to feed her she'd still lost weight. Lucy was told that, if she'd lost weight by the next session, she would be hospitalised. I was told that it was my duty, as a parent, to ensure that she didn't lose weight. This may sound harsh but I think it helped in a way by forcing me to feed her even though, by this time, it was so very difficult. I only wish they'd shown me how to feed my child or what to expect during the process.

After that we saw CAMHS twice a week as well as appointments with the psychologist, dietician and our own GP. There was very little in the way of practical help for me from the CAMHS team; their focus was on Lucy. They would give Lucy hand-outs and reading material about body dysmorphia or healthy eating, but it was pointless: she wouldn't even look at them.

Lucy's nurse told me that, although it was possible to recover from anorexia, on average it could take between six and eight years. In other words, I should expect a long drawn out process. I couldn't believe what I was hearing. Good grief, that would put my daughter into her *twenties* before she got well. What about her teenage years? What about school? University? All those years that are so very important? I decided there and then that I didn't want this for my daughter. I would do everything in my power to ensure she recovered within *months* rather than *years*.

However I wasn't encouraged when Lucy spent every therapy session staring at the floor, refusing to participate. By this stage her brain functioning was so poor that she just wasn't capable of engaging with anyone. CAMHS didn't seem to share the urgency I felt and seemed resigned to the fact Lucy would need to be hospitalised. They told me not to push her too fast and that it had to be her choice to get better. She had to "want" to get better. I disagreed. I didn't feel she was capable of making any rational choices. The only consistent piece of information I'd found so far had said that the earlier the treatment, the better the outcome. So I felt as if I was racing against the clock. If I waited for Lucy to "want" to get better it could eat up months or even years of her valuable life. I wasn't prepared to wait.

I got the feeling that CAMHS really didn't expect me to be able to re-feed Lucy at home. They kept saying that very few parents are able to do this. But I'd think, well, that's hardly surprising if parents aren't being *shown* how to re-feed their child or given any support outside the treatment sessions. If parents fail, then why on earth isn't someone being dispatched into the home to show them how to do it? It just seemed crazy that this kind of support wasn't being offered. But whenever I asked what help was available they'd look at me and say: "Nothing that we're aware of." Looking back, having some coaching and coping techniques would have made all the difference. So much so that I often wonder whether all those hours of therapy, talking about feelings, health implications and nutrition were a total waste of NHS time and money. Lucy, too, could have done with some coping strategies of her own. But, as far as I am aware, this wasn't happening. We felt so alone.

Initially I tried to keep family life going as near normal as possible. I went to work and Lucy went to school. Inevitably by the time I got to work she'd text me begging to be picked up. She just couldn't cope and neither could I. Eventually we were both so exhausted that I took her out of school and asked for some time off work. This way I could devote all my time to getting her to eat and gain weight.

After that it was a constant cycle of cooking, feeding, shopping, hospital appointments and talking - or just being there to comfort and distract her. Thankfully, her school was very supportive and sent work home but to be honest it was pointless, she wasn't able to concentrate on anything.

Her depression deepened and in her darkest moments she would tell me how frightened she was and that she didn't deserve to live. She was scared she would take her own life. She left her diaries lying where she knew I would find them. They were filled with details of the harm she was inflicting on herself and of self-hatred and loathing. They were truly horrifying but at least they helped me to keep her safe which I'm sure, deep down, was her intention. I am certain that those diaries were a cry for help.

As a family we watched her 24/7 ensuring that all medicines and sharp objects were kept out of her way. I slept with her every night and she was never alone. CAMHS wanted to prescribe antidepressants but Lucy refused and CAMHS felt it was morally wrong to force her. It really was a living nightmare and, without question, the worst time of my life.

I bought books, read articles and watched online videos, trying to collect as much knowledge as I could. I rang and emailed people. Then, fortunately, I found the F.E.A.S.T. website and the ATDT forum. I'm so glad I did. Immediately I realised my instincts had been correct; that Lucy needed to eat - and that she needed to do it quickly.

The relief was enormous. At last there were people who had walked in my shoes and really understood how I felt. They had answers for all my questions and there was always someone there to listen to me, day or night. For the first time I felt as if I wasn't alone.

I realised that what we were going through was not only normal during re-feeding but a pretty typical reaction and that we mustn't give up. We just had to keep going and things would get better. There was so much helpful advice based on families' own experiences together with suggestions and ideas plus lots of genuine, caring, heartfelt sympathy. It gave me the motivation I needed.

I carried on re-feeding; by now I had plenty of high calorie meal ideas. I knew all the items with the highest calories in every major supermarket! I even sneaked extra calories into Lucy's meals. Adding double cream, cheese or butter to everything became the norm. I kept Lucy out of the kitchen and she stopped questioning what was going into her meals. Very, very slowly her resistance began to weaken. I think that, once she realised that I wouldn't back down and that losing weight wasn't an option, she came to the conclusion that I was more determined than the eating disorder. She could see there was little point in fighting and, to be honest, I think she found it almost a relief. She began to gain weight and mealtimes became more manageable. The anxiety was still there, but as long as we didn't focus on the food and distracted her afterwards, she could cope and so could we.

Two months later she was well over half-way to her target weight. In fact she felt well enough to return to school for one or two lessons a day. She was fortunate to have a really good, close group of friends who stood by her and kept her "in the loop". They were, and still are, an enormous support. Her teachers, too, helped her to catch up by providing extra support. Gradually she increased the amount of time spent at school and started socialising once more. My husband and I began to see glimpses of our wonderful daughter again.

We are still in the process of re-feeding. There have been a few ups and downs along the way but Lucy is almost at her target weight and things are so much better. Since returning to school full-time, together with an increase in her weight, we have noticed something else significant: Lucy is enjoying life more and doing normal teenage things. Her concentration has also improved and she's catching up with school work. Eating is much easier and nowadays she recognises just how ill she was - however she remembers very little of what happened; she finds it all so very hazy.

We got our daughter through this. It was hell, but we did it. I am not super-human in any way. I am just a normal, common-or-garden mum. But Lucy's anorexia brought out the fighter in me and, if the truth be told, I attribute this to the ATDT forum and the amazing support I received there, and still receive to this day. I would not have been able to fight my daughter's illness without their encouragement or belief in me.

Our daughter is back with us and we are very hopeful that, in time, she will fully recover and lead an independent and happy, normal life, free from eating disorders. And she's back with us *months* after being diagnosed, not *years* as we were led to expect. Again, I put this down to the knowledge and support I received from F.E.A.S.T. and the ATDT forum. This, and the prompt action by our GP right at the start which I am convinced saved my daughter's life.

MY TIPS:

Keep a record of height and weight as your child grows up. My records ended when my children were pre-school. As a result it made it very difficult to identify a potential problem but also to set an accurate target weight. Growing bodies shouldn't be losing weight - watch out for a plateau with an increase in height. Don't make an issue of weighing; just make it a regular thing and start when your children are little, like measuring their height or going to the dentist.

Know what to look out for. Be aware that severe weight loss is not always the first thing that's noticed, and indeed not always present. Usually, by that time, things have been going on for quite a while and, anyway, it's easily disguised. The first symptoms of my daughter's anorexia were anxiety, depression, panic attacks, low self-esteem and perfectionism. As her illness progressed we noticed extreme sensitivity to cold, speaking very quietly, irritability, obsessive behaviours, an increase in exercise and only wanting to eat healthy foods. We didn't notice how severe her weight loss was until we took her to the GP for diagnosis.

Keep communicating with your child. Don't assume it's "just their age". Teenagers are notoriously private. Keep reminding them that you are there for them. Don't dismiss their problems. Whilst their problems may seem trivial to you they are very real and relevant to them. Be sympathetic, not judgemental.

Trust your gut instincts, you know your child better than anyone. Don't be fobbed off if you believe there is a problem. Keep fighting.

Act quickly and don't put it off. It doesn't get any easier the longer you leave it.

Don't expect friends and family to understand what it's like to live with a child who has anorexia or how serious it is. Most people still think they can just "snap out of it", as though they have chosen this for themselves. Educate them; their support will be a great help.

Read, read, read - learn everything you can. Some of it will be useful, some not. Use what you need and what is helpful in your situation. Be realistic about how hard re-feeding can be. Know the pitfalls to avoid and the loopholes to close. If you are fortunate to have a good support network around you - use it. If you are re-feeding at home, be prepared to ask for some time off work. Accept that for a period of time your life may revolve around your child's illness.

Finally… Have faith that your child will recover!

Glenda's story

"Through the ATDT forum I realised that the re-feeding nightmare... the long periods sitting around the table, the awful atmosphere, the anger, the crying and all those things... were normal."

Looking back I can recognise the early warning signs. Cecily was always very controlled about what and how much she ate. She never overindulged. She was never very adventurous. And once, when she was young, I remember her wishing she had a zip in her tummy to put food in so that she didn't have to taste it.

Also, when Cecily was transitioning from primary school to high school, I remember writing on the medical form that I was concerned about her eating. I also remember voicing my concerns to some friends that I was worried that Cecily might have the potential to develop an eating disorder.

When she was 12, Cecily became vegetarian. I agreed, provided she still ate fish to provide her with protein as she didn't like cheese. But within the year she was back to eating meat.

Cecily was always very clever, very academic and also very musically talented. She was always keen to participate in sport, especially climbing. Although she had been a quiet, book-loving child with only a few friends at primary school, I didn't realise that her self-confidence was so low. But once she began at high school (a different school from her friends) she transformed into someone who got involved in lots of extracurricular activities: sport, music, debating and so on. I think the debating surprised us most because it takes a lot of guts to stand up and speak in front of an audience.

In retrospect I think Cecily was reinventing herself. She'd gone from being the top academic pupil at our local primary school to being one of many very clever girls at the high school. Looking back she may have found this difficult to deal with and may have put herself under too much pressure to achieve and strive to be the best.

It's strange, but all the things I used to admire, I now see as a curse and part of her emerging eating disorder: the drive to be a high achiever, a perfectionist and to be involved in as much as possible. To me, these are all part and parcel of the anorexia mind set.

Whilst on holiday in Italy in July 2011, I remember 14-year old Cecily asking me whether I knew anyone with an eating disorder. Initially I said that, no I didn't, but later I told her that her aunt had suffered from anorexia for three decades. Certainly I never really understood the extent of the aunt's problem. I always wondered why she didn't just eat, why she was always so standoffish and why she would avoid family occasions. I thought it was a choice. These days, however, I know that it wasn't; she was - and still is - being driven by the illness.

Cecily was just 15 when I began to feel uncomfortable about a few things. She had always been a big milk drinker, but during one particular week we seemed to have a glut of milk. I noticed that Cecily was drinking mostly water. The milk was mainly untouched.

Then, on her sister's birthday, she refused to have a slice of birthday cake. We went out to an Italian restaurant for a birthday meal and Cecily complained about the greasiness of the garlic bread. She ordered a child's portion and refused to have a dessert. She'd never been overly enthusiastic about food, but it still seemed a bit peculiar.

That same weekend she and her friend came in late from a school disco. I offered both girls a slice of cake. Her friend tucked in, but - again - Cecily refused. It just felt odd.

Increasingly I noticed that she wasn't taking her usual morning snack to school. Often after school she'd be involved in a plethora of extracurricular activities and I'd pick her up late. I remember that autumn in particular. She would be absolutely ravenous by the time she got into the car. She'd text me beforehand asking me to bring in some food, so I'd take in a banana or a muffin. But I just assumed that all these activities had made her hungry when, in fact, it was because she'd scarcely eaten anything during the day.

I quizzed her about the morning snack. But she said everyone was too busy to eat snacks these days and so I just accepted this as fact. Never mind, I thought, at least she's getting a solid hot meal at lunchtime. It was only when a couple of her friends phoned me to say they were worried about Cecily's eating that I realised she was just having soup and a roll for lunch. Later she ditched the roll altogether.

Another thing that bothered me was that Cecily had always had a great relationship with her dad. They'd walk to the bus stop every morning, chatting away. But for a couple of months she'd been noticeably "off" and really critical of him. We put it down to adolescence, teenage sort of stuff.

Also, on the days when she didn't have any extracurricular activities, she would get home and go straight up to her room whereas, before, she'd come into the kitchen and we'd have a nice chat over a cuppa. Her moods began to change, too. One minute she'd be very clingy and weepy, wanting to sit on my knee a lot, and the next she'd be cold, detached and snappy. It was so unlike her to have huge mood swings. But, again, I thought it was just adolescence. Or at least I did until one day when I saw her standing at the kitchen sink getting a glass of water. She was literally shaking with hunger, yet she was filling up on water instead of food. She was drinking an awful lot of water. I began to wonder whether something else was going on and it wasn't just Cecily being a grouchy, fussy teenager.

Like many families, we had no idea what Cecily's weight was. I don't think she'd been weighed since she was a toddler; healthy children just aren't weighed as a matter of course in the UK. We didn't know her height, either. And the acronym "BMI" meant little to us. But she looked thinner, she looked paler and she was freezing cold all the time. She just couldn't get enough layers on. The house was so hot it was like a furnace, yet she'd shake with cold.

Very soon I began to put two and two together. I thought about the eating disordered aunt again. Indeed one day it suddenly struck me that Cecily was looking more and more like this aunt. I was horrified. I knew I had to talk to Cecily. The trouble was, how was I going to go about it? It was such a scary subject to broach. My stomach was churning and it was quite frightening to approach her. When I eventually did, she was in total denial; she just said it was all about her wanting to be "healthy". I explained my concerns to her - that I thought she was looking thinner and that she was always cold and pale, and also that her friends had spoken to me. But she denied anything was wrong.

I wouldn't say Cecily was happy to come to the GP but she didn't resist. I said: "Well, why don't we go to the GP just so he can rule out an eating disorder?" I told her the GP might say she's fine. I even told her that, if things improved after the weekend, then I would cancel the appointment.

Things didn't improve. So, just a few days before Christmas, I went with Cecily to the GP. I was quite happy to wait outside, but I think Cecily wanted me to be there, so in I went. I voiced my concerns and the GP asked Cecily a few questions. What did she like to eat? (Answer: "Salad.") Did she think there was a problem? (Answer: "No, not really.") How were things at school? (Answer: "Fine.") The GP weighed her and told her to come back in three weeks' time.

That Christmas was very tense, especially as we had family with us. We didn't want to spoil their Christmas with our concerns, especially as everyone was permanently worried about the aunt with anorexia. Normally Cecily would have loved chatting and joking with her granddad, but that Christmas she stayed in her room a lot and didn't interact much. She was constantly cold, in spite of having the radiator up at full blast and sitting against it wearing a fleece with the hood up. By now I was getting really concerned. What had happened to the normal chirpy Cecily we'd been so used to? It was Christmas, yet she was just so emotionless. It was truly awful to watch.

Cecily sat her GCSE mock examinations in early January and, despite finding it hard to focus and concentrate on revision at this point, she gained a string of A grades. Then, in mid-January, we returned to the GP who again asked questions about her diet, how she felt and so on. Cecily was also weighed. I was horrified to see that she'd lost three kilos in three weeks.

The GP asked Cecily if she felt she needed help to which Cecily replied that she didn't think she did. I remember my stomach churning, thinking that I wasn't going to have any say in the matter. Fortunately the GP thought that it might be a good thing to put forward a referral. Within a few days we received an appointment at our local CAMHS unit.

At that time I had no idea what "CAMHS" was. I didn't know who we were being referred to until the letter came through the post. Also, I didn't know whether it was usual for an appointment to come through so quickly or whether I should be worried. I just didn't know anything at all. Well, you don't, do you? I felt as if I was entering a whole new world with a whole new vocabulary packed with puzzling acronyms.

At CAMHS we met with a psychiatrist and a nurse. After talking about our family life, Cecily's childhood and our concerns, Cecily was weighed and measured, and diagnosed with anorexia. Over the next few days the different treatment options were discussed, and we opted for FBT (Family-Based Treatment).

Over the previous weeks I had spent many stomach churning sleepless nights researching anorexia and how to treat it, and FBT kept coming up as the best evidence-based approach. I hadn't expected it to be offered and so was surprised and relieved that this was our recommended route.

Through FBT we managed to get Cecily's weight back up to the level it was when I first took her to see the GP. There wasn't a meal plan as such, it was just a case of having to eat what we ate; Cecily had to have three meals and three snacks a day. It was tough, with lots of long periods sitting around the dinner table and lots of crying and refusing to eat. We felt as if we were on a perpetual knife-edge, constantly treading on eggshells, terrified of setting her off by saying or doing the wrong thing. But, bit by bit, we managed it.

Initially I trusted Cecily to be eating her dinner at school and then we switched to a packed lunch. But she began to lose weight. I discovered she wasn't eating her lunch and was throwing away her snack. So I began to go into school every break and lunchtime and sit with her while she ate.

Every week we'd all meet with the family therapist. Cecily's sister was invited along, too, but that didn't last long because her sister was fed up with missing out on school and we couldn't really see much benefit in her being there.

At the CAMHS sessions we'd discuss what had happened that week and voice any concerns. It was very much focused on weight and the reasons why Cecily might have lost or gained that weight, and what we could do to keep the momentum moving forward or stop any losses, so, yes, I did feel that we were getting support. But Cecily never, ever wanted to be part of that. To be honest, I don't think at that point that she would have wanted to be part of any treatment we had chosen. But at least she was going along to the sessions.

Then over the summer Cecily had a relapse. She'd worked with us in the lead up to the GCSE examinations and had put on a certain amount of weight but she was by no means back to her pre-anorexic weight. But after the exams she got stuck. Then when the summer holidays came she just went downhill. She literally stopped eating.

I'd just found the Around The Dinner Table forum. Through this I realised that the re-feeding nightmare we'd gone through over the last few months... the long periods sitting around the table, the awful atmosphere, the anger, the crying and all those things... were normal. I only wish I'd found it five months previously! I also realised that the way we, as parents, were feeling was normal as well.

But when Cecily stopped eating and began to go downhill again I was devastated. It had taken so much effort, so much work and it had had such an impact on everybody in the family - and now, with this relapse, I felt as if we were back to Square One. I can't tell you how disheartening that felt.

Eventually Cecily was admitted to a specialist eating disorders unit as a day patient. I'd phoned CAMHS one morning and said: "I can't stand this anymore. I can't stand to see her eating a teaspoon of Weetabix" because, at this point, she was just eating small bits and pieces. So they referred her to the unit.

Cecily was there for about six weeks. She came home every night, but all the eating was done at the unit. Gradually meals were introduced at home: first breakfast, then the odd evening meal and finally lunch.

They managed to halt the downward spiral and put it into reverse, so there was a slight improvement by the time she was discharged. Cecily wasn't recovered by any stretch of the imagination and certainly not physically better, although she was gaining weight very slowly.

CAMHS felt the FBT wasn't working. Cecily was just too strong-willed and independent. Actually, just after she was discharged, we began to have some real support on the eating front. Someone from CAMHS would go into school and sit with her while she had her lunch. I only wish we'd had this kind of support a long time before.

I also wish I'd found the ATDT forum much sooner. By the time I read through the relevant posts, posted questions of my own and discovered all the right things to say and do, it was almost too late for us. Up to that point no-one had told us things like "food is medicine". No-one had shown us how to coach her through a meal.

But I had to trust Cecily to have her own snacks at school. This was quite scary because, you know, it's not normal to have to control your 16-year old daughter's eating but at the same time suddenly giving her this independence was scary. What if she didn't eat these snacks?

Now, some eight months on from being discharged from the unit,

Cecily has been given total independence on the eating front apart from evening meals which I prepare. She's still seeing CAMHS but right now she's in a rut. Around Christmastime she stopped sharing some information with us, so we don't know what her weight is but I'd hazard a guess that she hasn't gained anything since December.

Cecily will be 17 in the summer. And of course because of her age she has certain legal rights; she doesn't have to share information with us if she doesn't want to. But the good news is that she keeps going to CAMHS. She could so easily refuse and we wouldn't be able to do anything about it. The trouble is that, now, she thinks she is recovered. Yet she still goes to CAMHS so there's a bit of anomaly there because I guess if she really felt she was recovered then she wouldn't go!

But, for the present, no-one - neither us nor CAMHS - seems to be able to get Cecily out of this rut and I worry that she could be stuck for some time. Not knowing her weight has actually done her a huge favour because I used to focus on the weight quite a bit and now I don't, simply because I don't know what it is. But there are other behaviours that have become more apparent now. For instance the other week I found a couple of receipts in her pocket from the gym.

Sometimes she almost makes me believe that this is her and this is the way she's going to be - and then when I find things like this I think: "Well this isn't normal; it's not normal to go to the gym and fib about it or hide food under your bed because you don't want to eat it." It takes me back to when she'd hide food in her pocket at suppertime or pass food to the dog under the table.

Actually, thinking about it… Not once during the whole of her eating disorder, with the exception of a couple of times while she was in the unit in the summer, has she admitted there is a problem. And I simply don't have any leverage. I can't use the threat of her having to go back into the unit if she doesn't turn things around because her weight isn't low enough to qualify for admission. So we're stuck. But I'm coming to terms with the fact that this is where we're going to be until I can come up with a solution to nudge things forward again.

The things that keep giving us hope are, firstly, that we got Cecily in front of CAMHS so quickly and, secondly, that as her family we will never give up on her. We will always be there for her no matter what.

Meanwhile, I keep reading and researching, and talking to other carers via the ATDT forum and at various eating disorders conferences, so I feel armed to deal with this awful illness. And we will deal with it, maybe not next week or even next month. But hopefully very soon we will find a way to guide Cecily onto the next stage of recovery.

Sandra's story

"My son's anorexia helped me realise what is important in life. Many things seem so trivial compared to what we've been through. You see things in a different light. And that is good in a bizarre kind of way."

I often wonder what triggered Jack's food restriction. Was it because he'd recently started at secondary school and his best friend had gone elsewhere? Did he feel a bit vulnerable and lonely without his friend? Or was it to do with his grandfather passing away shortly before things began to go downhill? You just don't know, do you?

One incident stands out, though. Jack was 13 and we'd gone to visit my husband's family in New York. The first comment that my sister-in-law made when we got off the plane was: "Wow, you are so thin, Jack!" Then one morning Jack got out of bed and promptly fainted. I wondered if it might be the heat or something. But ten minutes later he stood up and passed out again. For a fleeting moment I thought: "Something isn't right here." But then he went downstairs, got some breakfast and we all carried on as normal.

Then my in-laws began to remark about Jack's appearance; that he seemed to have lost quite a bit of weight. Well, his dad and I hadn't noticed. You don't tend to notice gradual changes when you're with your child all the time. So I put it to the back of my mind.

Back in the UK, Jack announced that he was going vegetarian. At first I was delighted. Jack had always been fussy about vegetables and this seemed to be a move in the opposite direction. I was pleased that he was so keen to eat more healthily. It didn't strike me as odd at all, not with all the stuff in the media and on the telly about eating healthily, getting your five a day and so on.

So I willingly bought him vegetarian and healthy eating cookbooks. I just couldn't get over the fact that he was now readily eating vegetables! Even when he started to buy fat-free cook books, it didn't dawn on me that there could be a potential eating disorder looming.

But then I noticed he was beginning to have hardly anything for breakfast. I thought: "Well this is a bit odd because he's always loved breakfast." Not once did I ever think it might be an eating disorder. You don't think about eating disorders when you have a boy.

Then my husband went away on business for three weeks. During this time things went from bad to worse. It was just awful. Jack refused to eat anything. He'd come home about 4 o'clock from school looking terrible. I'd found out from his friend's mum that he hadn't eaten anything all day, even though he was claiming to have had a big school lunch. He was also starting to mention to his friends that he felt great, almost euphoric, when he didn't eat anything. He'd get home and say that he was really tired and cold (it was minus-eight outside and of course he'd been running on empty since the morning). So he'd say he was going to have a shower and go straight to bed. At suppertime I'd go up to his room but he wouldn't wake up. Looking back, I think he must have been pretending to be asleep.

My husband came back from the business trip, took one look at Jack and said: "What on earth has been happening?" Again, because I'd been with Jack every day, I guess I hadn't noticed the change. But his dad picked up on it straight away. It just goes to show how quickly things can go downhill in such a short space of time.

Mood-wise Jack was becoming very withdrawn. He'd also been isolating himself from his friends since the summer. And he had this thing about sweets. One of his friends said he'd give him £250 if he didn't eat sweets for two years and Jack kept going on about what a great idea this was, so obviously this was going on in his mind as well.

Just before Christmas I took Jack to see the GP and told him I was concerned about the weight loss and all the other things that were going on. The GP said that it was probably just a phase, maybe due to stress at school. He asked us to come back after the Christmas holidays for a review by which time hopefully things would have improved.

They didn't. Over Christmas, things just went from bad to worse. In fact it was horrendous. My parents came over and Jack refused to eat most of the food that was put in front of him. Everyone was in tears at the Christmas dinner table. It was awful.

In desperation I phoned NHS Direct to ask for advice because, by this time, Jack was refusing to have even a glass of water. They put me through to a psychiatric nurse who talked to me for about an hour. But it's all very well talking, but none of it was really helping me. Another night I phoned them up, spoke to a doctor and told her that he wouldn't even drink a glass of water. She asked Jack to get on the phone and eventually persuaded him to take a drink.

When our GP returned after the Christmas break she'd obviously seen a record of my calls to NHS Direct. She called me, said she'd refer Jack to CAMHS immediately and told us to take him down to A&E to get him physically checked over. At the hospital they took his pulse which was very low. He was also terribly cold. They hooked him up to an ECG monitor and wrapped him in a hypothermic blanket for a couple of hours. By now it was dawning on me just how desperately ill my son had become in such a short space of time. How could I have failed to notice this was happening?

Jack was then admitted to the children's ward where he stayed for about ten days while everyone kept a close eye on him. He was put on a complete bed rest order and monitored whenever he visited the bathroom. Shower times were limited, too. One of the male nurses was excellent as he had previously worked on a psychiatric ward and would often come over and chat to Jack and encourage him to eat more.

The good news is that Jack was eating on the ward, although there were certain things he'd refuse to have, but at least he was getting three meals a day inside him. To illustrate how ill he was, though, the mere thought of seeing the snack trolley trundle along the ward made him black out. I never did find out if this was fake or not but the nurses took his blood pressure and it had dipped. As a result of being on the ward his weight did increase; not a huge amount but it did increase a bit. Meanwhile the CAMHS team came into the hospital and met with us to talk about a treatment plan for Jack.

Back home, Jack didn't want to eat. On the very first day I remember him walking up the stairs, stopping half-way up, taking a picture off the wall and threatening to throw it at me if I made him eat lunch. So I phoned CAMHS who said: "Well, it's only one meal that he's missed."

We saw CAMHS twice a week: a session with a psychologist and another with a psychiatrist who would weigh him, take his blood pressure and pulse. Meanwhile my brain had gone into a kind of autopilot. We just went into the sessions and did what was required to get his weight back up. I was still working at this time. So I'd leave work, pick him up from school and bring him home to eat his lunch and then take him back to school. This way I could be sure of him eating something in the middle of the day. Getting all those calories into him was just so much hard work, though. But his weight did begin to creep up. He started eating meat, and having milk on his cereal which I was really pleased about.

Mentally, however, it took a few months for things to improve. Meanwhile, although I was happy with the treatment he was getting from the psychologist, I wasn't too enamoured with the psychiatrist who tended to treat Jack as if he were a naughty little boy for not eating. But we are fortunate in that Jack went along to the treatment sessions quite willingly. He'd take along a diary every week to show them what he'd been eating, that kind of thing.

We saw CAMHS for about a year. Things went well. But then they made the mistake of asking Jack if he felt he needed to carry on with treatment and, of course, he said no. So he was discharged - and ever since we've been kind of managing things by ourselves.

But it was a tough time. Like most families, I guess, I looked around the internet for advice and information. That was when I found Bev Mattocks' blog: *AnorexiaBoyRecovery*. Through this I discovered F.E.A.S.T. and the Around The Dinner Table forum, and built up some really great supportive relationships with the other parents there, especially those from the UK. At the time the forum was a Godsend. I don't use it so much now that Jack is doing so well. But, looking back, I don't think I could have got through all this without the help and support I found there. I wasn't getting any emotional or behind-the-scenes support from CAMHS.

These days Jack still likes to have a routine and he still gets quite uptight about certain things which is something we need to work on. But he does have exams coming up, so it's probably best to wait until those are over before knuckling down and working away at it all again. He's studying hard and did very well in his mock exams.

His weight is steady and so is his mood. Sometimes there's a bit of a dip and you think, "Oh no, he's heading back into the abyss" but, in general, he seems fine. He's happy to go out for meals, although you'd never find him going for the fish'n'chips option; it's usually a curry or something like that. But, on the whole, he doesn't want to talk about the eating disorder.

I'm still getting used to being off the "autopilot" I was in for the whole period. I remember getting very depressed last summer, lying on the couch and not wanting to do anything. Jack got quite upset, telling me I wasn't being myself and wanting to know what was wrong. I took time off work and went down to see my parents. I also took some time off with stress. I just wasn't functioning well. This was odd, because by then Jack was so much better. I think it was almost like a kind of post-traumatic stress thing. I think that, during the worst of the eating disorder, you're so busy frantically trying to tackle the problem that it's not until afterwards that it suddenly hits you. For instance, for some time afterwards, I'd wake up in the early hours with my mind racing and I'd have panic attacks for no reason at all.

Some days I do wonder if we'll ever be completely rid of the legacy of the eating disorder or whether it will be with us forever. I will always feel that we have to keep an eye on things to make sure it doesn't creep back in because I know how easy it can be for young people to relapse.

On the plus side, however, it's helped me realise what is important in life. When something crops up at work, for example, I don't worry as much as I used to do. Many things just seem so trivial compared to what we've been through. You see things in a different light. And that is good in a bizarre kind of way.

Shirley's story

"A teacher said: 'Here we are, talking about academic achievements. But, for Rebecca, walking into school every day is an achievement compared to these other students.' That was so lovely. Rebecca nearly cried. And so did I!"

When did it all start? When did things change? When did it stop being my normal, beautiful daughter having a few issues with being a teenager and begin to be the descent into full-blown anorexia? It's something that always puzzles me. I don't think I can pinpoint any particular moment when I could say: "Yesterday my child was fine; today she has anorexia." You see, this illness creeps up on everyone so very gradually.

With hindsight it's easy to look back and wonder if it was the spring of 2011 when Rebecca was 16 and studying for her GCSE examinations. Or did it begin even earlier than this? From around October 2010 onwards she'd been getting more and more depressed. By Easter I was sufficiently concerned to take her to the GP who referred her to a counselling service. (In the event that never happened.)

Rebecca had never been a fussy eater; she'd always eaten well. She didn't eat meat, but we'd always been a vegetarian family. Also, Rebecca was very slim, slimmer than most of her friends. But, to us, this was normal because she'd always been this way.

So, looking back, it's really hard to work out when the change took place. But after Easter 2011 I gradually began to notice a change in her eating habits. One morning I said to her: "Why are you cutting up grapes?" She had whittled her breakfast down to just fruit which she would cut up into lots of tiny pieces and proceed to eat slowly with a small fork. I thought: "This isn't normal."

I had a word with my best friend who said: "But she looks fine!" And, to be truthful, she did look okay. We'd just been swimming and my friend said: "Look, Shirley, Rebecca is absolutely fine. But if you're worried, then it mightn't be a bad idea to take her to the GP?"

I knew something was wrong, but I didn't know what. As a mother I think you sense when something is up - a slight change in your child's mannerisms or something as simple as an expression you don't recognise. Also, eating was becoming more and more difficult. Then Rebecca began to cut out carbs and fats. But it still didn't register with me. I still wasn't thinking: "Oh my God, she's got an eating disorder!" And I'm a trained nurse. But I really didn't recognise an emerging eating disorder when I saw it.

Rebecca would eat, but it would take her ages. I can still see her, sitting out in the garden with a baked potato and salad, eating it bit by bit. She'd also begun to reduce the size of her portions and was slowly cutting back on what she would eat. By June 2011 she was down to just three small meals a day: mainly fruit, vegetables, fish and sweet potato. She was also exercising more and more.

As a parent you have a gut instinct when things aren't quite right. So sometime in mid-June I rang our GP. I specifically asked to speak to a young GP who I knew Rebecca liked. I told her that I knew Rebecca was depressed, but I was also really worried about the eating. I asked if perhaps I could send her into see the GP under the pretext of something else. She was taking medication for heavy periods, so the GP agreed to call Rebecca in for a "review".

Rebecca didn't want me to come with her. But the GP was very good and phoned me back afterwards. She said: "Yes, you are right. I've weighed her and her weight has gone down. I think we need to refer her to CAMHS." It was a relief.

During the summer holidays Rebecca got worse and worse. And

meanwhile we were still waiting for the CAMHS appointment which wasn't being treated as urgent. Eventually an appointment came through for mid-August. But we were overseas visiting family, so I had to change it to later in the month. We never did get that other appointment to see the counsellor about Rebecca's depression but I guess that, now we were going to see CAMHS, it didn't really matter.

Well, the overseas trip was awful. At the time I didn't realise I should be insisting that she ate; I just let her eat what she wanted, when she felt like it while she continued to lose weight. I really regret this in hindsight. I remember my mum saying: "Why don't you sit with her and make her eat?" But I just let her get on with her tweaked eating regime.

One day Rebecca decided to get drunk with her cousins, on an empty stomach. The police rang me to say she'd collapsed. Later on in the holiday I remember taking her to buy some jeans. She'd shrunk to a children's size (which thrilled her). Everyone had started to notice by this point saying: "She's not eating…" And everyone could see she was getting weaker.

In that space of time between visiting the GP and coming back from overseas, Rebecca had lost an awful lot of weight. Up to then it had been very gradual. But it's surprising how quickly they deteriorate once the rollercoaster gets going. She'd also started to increase her fluid intake quite drastically and was exercising non-stop.

But I still thought that once we got her to CAMHS everything would be alright. It would be a case of a quick diagnosis, some swift treatment and it would all be over and done with. Job done. That's what I really thought at the time.

So it came as a shock when it wasn't a "quick fix".

I said to CAMHS: "Has she got anorexia?"

The response was: "I think so…"

I said: "Well she either has or she hasn't, really."

The trouble is I guess it's not easy to diagnose an eating disorder; it's not like pregnancy, anaemia or something. You can't just take a blood or urine sample and you know what you're dealing with.

I asked the psychiatrist what was going to happen next. She said they'd "watch her for a bit".

One day I went up to Rebecca's bedroom and was horrified to find it covered in post-it notes with the words "pig", "ugly pig" and so on scrawled on them. She had even stuck them into her vest to ensure that she didn't forget what an "ugly pig" she was. She wrote "pig" on her mirror, in her diary, everywhere. She bought socks with pigs on them. It was heart-breaking.

By this stage I'd found F.E.A.S.T. and read the website through from start to finish. I'd also joined the ATDT forum where I'd posted up my concerns and chatted with other families. And the more I found out about eating disorders, the stranger it seemed that - at no point - had CAMHS told me I needed to feed my child. I find that really scary.

The psychiatrist said she'd set up an appointment with a psychologist for a couple of weeks' time. In the meantime she suggested that I "back off" a bit. She told me I should trust my daughter to be able to eat, even at school. But I knew she wasn't eating at school because she was losing weight.

I was also instructed to leave Rebecca alone after a meal. Now, again, I knew that after meals Rebecca would go off and exercise like mad. Star jumps and press-ups were her favourite. And when she wasn't doing these she was banging her head against a wall. But the psychiatrist told me I needed to trust her and leave her alone after meals. And she told me this in front of Rebecca.

I can't begin to tell you how much aggro this caused when I completely ignored this and continued to feed my daughter as my maternal gut instinct told me to. Rebecca would say: "The psychiatrist told you to leave me alone!"

I would reply, "Well I'm not going to leave you alone" and I'd continue to feed her.

So Rebecca would say, "You should listen to her; she's the professional, not you" and it would escalate into a screaming argument. But I still wouldn't back down because after meals I knew she'd be jumping, jumping and jumping. And whenever I voiced my concerns about all the exercising, the CAMHS psychiatrist would tell me that it was "just a phase".

I said: "Surely not! Surely all this not eating and frantically doing star jumps and press-ups can't be 'just a phase'?" She was also drinking incredible volumes of water. I told the psychiatrist she was drinking at least six litres a day. But the response was: "Well, if she does the same every week, then it won't affect the weighing in any way." I was worried that drinking copious amounts of water could be dangerous!

Meanwhile Rebecca was drinking and drinking, exercising like mad and refusing to eat very much despite my efforts while I was being instructed to "back off".

However I carried on feeding her and managed to level out her weight. But the harder I tried to feed her, the harder the anorexia fought back. Being told to "back off" in front of my child made it a hundred times harder to get that life-giving food into her.

Then, one day, the psychiatrist went on leave and we saw another one who was much better. She took my concerns seriously and told me I should take Rebecca out of school. I thought: "Thank God for that!" I mean, my daughter was so weak she couldn't even walk through the CAMHS car park. This new psychiatrist told me to fetch my car and pick Rebecca up from the door. Oh, I was so very relieved... At last someone was agreeing with me that my daughter was very sick. And, because it was a professional saying all this, Rebecca seemed to be listening; it carried more clout. It was no longer "just my mum" ranting on.

So I told Rebecca she must stay at home, sit on the sofa and eat.

But then the original psychiatrist returned from leave and we found ourselves back in front of her.

I was alarmed when she said: "Now that Rebecca has had a week off, she can go back to school." So, as a compromise, I began to let her go for half days, picking her up at lunchtime.

Of course, by now, I'd had to leave work. I couldn't juggle caring for my daughter with working, especially the shifts I was expected to do as a nurse. Meals would take forever, too. Even something as "simple" as breakfast would take over an hour. Breakfast would run into snack time which would run into lunch which would run into afternoon snack time which would run into the evening meal which would run into the final snack for the day. It was one long hard slog.

Day after day after day.

And it wasn't just the daytime. At night I was often up there in her room, trying to stop her from exercising.

But despite all this she somehow managed to continue to lose weight. I felt like a failure; I just couldn't get that weight onto her. And it was mainly me that was having to deal with all this. I couldn't expect Rebecca's step dad to bear the brunt of things and, anyway, Rebecca would only eat with me.

I told CAMHS that I wanted Rebecca to be admitted to a unit for inpatient treatment. They weren't enthusiastic but the psychiatrist eventually said: "You might as well go and look around one, but I personally don't like those places."

I took Rebecca to visit a big hospital in the Midlands. They were in the process of setting up an adolescent eating disorders inpatient unit. A specialist nurse talked to Rebecca for an hour and then I talked with him for another hour, which was really great because he was actually taking me seriously. It was the very first time anyone had ever said to me: "You're actually doing okay." He told me he thought the way I was managing Rebecca's eating "was fantastic".

"Really?" I said, surprised. "Nobody's ever told me that!"

He said Rebecca needed to be admitted. So I said that if she was going to be admitted then it was probably best if she went in sooner rather than later. She was admitted the next day.

Initially we thought she was going to be there for three months. In the event it was eight months before she came out, in summer 2012.

I was dreading her coming out. She'd already been home for a few weekends which had been disastrous.

On one occasion she tried to climb out of a window. On another, she ran off, sat in the middle of a field and just screamed and screamed. There was always some drama going on.

Meanwhile she made friends with another girl in the unit and this girl said to her: "You know what? Our mums are never going to give up. We may as well eat."

So she came home.

The problem was that after eight months of hospitalisation she'd become institutionalised. She'd got very used to the rigid structure and the meal planning, because they had a three-week rotating menu which they were allowed to choose themselves. So I had to do menu planning with her, starting with her final week in hospital so she knew in advance what she was going to be eating when she came out.

Since she's been out, she's always eaten. We're also working on helping her to socialise, get back into society and not "be a patient" any longer. She emerged from hospital very immature for her age. Thankfully we had the summer holidays to work on all of this. But getting her de-institutionalised wasn't easy. When she first came out she even asked me for permission to go to the toilet!

But, really, these days she eats relatively well, although she needs to know in advance what we're planning to eat and she can't eat on her own. Her weight is fine, too. On occasions she's lost the odd bit, but she knows she needs to put it on again. Only the other night she said to me: "Mum, I know I've got to gain a bit of weight. What's the best way to do it?"

She is really brave and I thought that was lovely.

Rebecca is still a little depressed. She is still on medication for it. She's had to go down a year at school because she lost a whole year and the hospital schooling wasn't great. She's with younger children and that's suiting her, actually. Just the last few months or so she's started to socialise more which is also good. She's going on school trips, too.

But it's been slow.

The other week Rebecca and I went along to parents' evening at school. Well, I felt like crying - what a contrast to last time! I remember back then she wouldn't touch me, she wouldn't talk to me, she would barely acknowledge me for months. Yet here we were having a laugh and a joke at parents' evening. Meanwhile she was getting glowing reports from the teachers. In one subject she'd achieved the highest mark ever in the school: one-hundred-per-cent. I was beside myself with pride.

Then another teacher said to us: "Here we all are, talking about academic achievements. But, for Rebecca, walking into this school every day is an achievement compared to these other students." That was so lovely. Rebecca nearly cried. And so did I!

To be honest, this meant more to us than the one-hundred-percent in the other subject.

So there we are. It's been a real slog, but Rebecca has made massive advances. She's been brilliant. As for me, well, as a parent you just get on with it, don't you? I still find myself having flashbacks and suddenly thinking: "Oh my God, that was horrendous!"

MY TIPS:

Seek help - as soon as you realise something is wrong as referral can sometimes take ages.

Start re-feeding whilst waiting for treatment, as treatment may not be the "magic wand" you expect it to be.

Educate yourself on eating disorders as much as possible, for example by visiting the F.E.A.S.T. website. Sort out your own support network - the ATDT forum is an excellent place to start. (See list of resources at the end of the book.)

Enlist the help of family and friends.

Realise that this is a serious condition which is going to take a long time to recover from.

Don't automatically assume that the healthcare professionals will be fully informed about eating disorders.

Remove the weighing scales from the house.

Search your child's room for food and signs of self-hatred, etc.

Stay with your child at all times whilst he/she eats and for at least an hour after each meal/snack to avoid possible purging.

Finally... be kind to yourself!!

POSTSCRIPT - by the author

A few weeks after talking to Shirley, I got this news: "Remember I told you about my daughter's 'pig phase'? Post-it notes with 'ugly fat pig' everywhere? On her vests, on her mirror and walls? Pig socks to remind her she was a greedy pig?

"Well, today Rebecca asked me to come to her room to look at something she was doing on the internet. On her mirror she had drawn a heart with 'I love you' inside it! I never would have thought that possible during the bad times, and there were many of them. During the really bad times sometimes I couldn't imagine things improving at all. It looked as if we were stuck for such a long time.

"Even after she came home from the unit, the anxieties were much the same. But slowly she started to trust me and trust the fact that my aim was not to make her fat. We are now closer than we were before the anorexia. Yes, we still have loads to work on. But I am so very, very proud of my daughter. She is incredibly brave and strong. So, please, everyone who is struggling, please keep fighting and don't lose hope!"

Finally...

At the beginning of this book I say: "I often wonder where we would be without the power of the internet." So I asked families the same question and this is what they came back with...

Martha, who suggested this topic would make an excellent postscript, said: "I, for one, am very sure that if I had followed our psychiatrist's treatment plan of 'They go up and down a few times until they get sick of doing it' my daughter would still be on the see-saw of multiple hospitalisations with no life of her own - particularly as she was one of the patients who plummeted to such a low weight. Instead I chose the slogan I'd learned about on the F.E.A.S.T. website: 'Food is Medicine'. I understood that my daughter had to learn to eat outside a hospital setting and I had to ensure she carried on with her normal life, hopes and dreams because this would ultimately drive her through it way more than hospitalisations with other sick patients."

Tanya contacted me immediately with: "Without the advances of the 'information super-highway' there is no doubt my daughter would still be languishing in anorexia. However, on the same note, there is enough misinformation to be dangerous as well. I strongly believe the strength of a parent's instinct is to search for the right answers as I did and I know so many others have done. Since we started on this journey two years ago, the work of parent advocates, clinicians and researchers has certainly helped to advance the availability of helpful eating disorder treatment information and the words 'evidence-based' are more readily found at the top of the pile of information when we search the internet for help.

"F.E.A.S.T. has become a force in itself with parent after parent and clinician after clinician referring families onto its website as a resource for accurate information; not to mention the strong source of support from the ATDT forum. Without the guidance and direction from other parents who have been through this nightmare illness I am not entirely certain where we would be now. The illness would have become so entrenched that, in fact, the firm recovery my daughter now enjoys may not have been possible without the valuable resource of the internet. Learning that this is a biologically-based illness and that the brain requires full nutrition for a long period for lasting recovery is what guided me to keep fighting the demon beast, never ever give up, and adopt a 'Life Stops until you EAT' approach; full stop! It just made sense and it works: one-hundred-per-cent nutrition one-hundred-per-cent of the time."

Eleanor, whose husband and mother contributed to this book, said: "Without the internet I wouldn't have had access to the contact form for Channel 4's *Supersize vs Superskinny* programme nor a wealth of information from the charity Beat. Where would I be today? Probably not sitting here in between my two beautiful babies and my wonderful husband!"

Dawn, however, saw the internet as a double-edged sword. "Yes the internet was a godsend for me in my desperate times. When I was feeling at the end of my tether, not knowing what to do next, I knew I could log onto the ATDT forum and either search for the answer to my question from the very knowledgeable friends at F.E.A.S.T. or just vent a little and know that there was always someone there to offer support and tell me to 'breathe'. I used the internet to research eating disorders, look for support networks and even used a route planner to tell me how to get to the hospital when my daughter was first admitted, and to A&E in a strange town when she was admitted after drinking cleaning fluids.

"On the flip side, however, my daughter used the internet to discover ways to hide her food or make people think she was eating.

She found websites that told her she was not yet thin enough and how guilty she should feel for eating that tiny morsel earlier in the day… that she should do 200 sit-ups to redeem herself or, worse, cut herself to feel the pain… So it's a double edged sword. The same resource that could have had a part in killing my daughter may also have played a part in saving her life."

On a similar topic, Tanya said: "I can't recall what my daughter did or did not find on the internet. However, having access to the internet contributed to Lauren becoming a walking encyclopaedia of calorie/fat content. You could perhaps argue, that whilst in the early days of re-feeding, we parents should restrict access to the internet in some way?"

Marianne said: "Without the power of the internet, although I feel we would still have received treatment and support from my daughter's treatment provider, I believe that we would be way behind in the recovery process. I would not have had the special support from my ATDT forum friends encouraging me and helping me to enable Lindy to eat. Nor would I have learned that I am part of the recovery process, not the cause of her eating disorder. So I'd probably be feeling powerless. But, thanks to the internet, I know that I am not!"

Shirley added: "Without the internet I would not have been able to access the information and support needed to guide my daughter to a safe recovery. I would not have had the courage to challenge the professionals. I certainly would not have received any support myself, which in turn has benefitted my daughter, Rebecca, immensely."

Caroline said: "At a time when our GP admitted she knew nothing about eating disorders (and neither did anyone else in the practice), the internet was the only place where I felt I could get any answers. As it happened, it ended up providing much more. Sifting through much of the nonsense takes time, but once I found an online community I trusted, they and the internet became a huge source of support, education and enablement."

Sandra contacted me with: "The internet has been invaluable

during my son's illness. Not only has it enabled me to find useful / official information on eating disorders but it has allowed me to connect to other families in the same boat. There is a down side, though, with all the pro-ana material available which could fuel the illness for many vulnerable young people."

Eva emailed to say: "Today, thanks to the internet, I offered a listening ear to yet another parent who is being subjected to every outdated belief you mention in your original question, and worse. If the clinicians involved are using the internet then it's failing to improve their knowledge or skills. So you ask this question on a day when I am both grateful for the internet and frustrated that it cannot guard against the failings of people or organisations."

Ruth came back to me with: "The internet proved to be our most important resource in finding out how we could help our daughter to overcome anorexia. When help was not forthcoming from healthcare professionals, we researched online and found Beat and their parents' help line. Amazon led us to several informative books on the subject of eating disorders. Later we found the F.E.A.S.T. website, containing information on the latest research, and the Around The Dinner Table Forum which gave us the opportunity to hear the stories of other families around the world who understood what we were going through and who could offer support."

Emma told me: "The internet helped me to see what was potentially wrong and gave me the courage to stand up with confidence to ask for - and then insist on - a specialist referral to our hospital of choice.

"Additionally, the internet then became my lifesaver when we were at our lowest ebb. Just reaching out daily to other parents on the ATDT forum who were in the same situation was so comforting because I had never felt so alone. The fact that life went on as normal right outside my front door was so surreal. I would look around me at the people hurrying about their daily lives and shout in my head: 'Don't you know what we are going through?! How can you just keep doing what you are doing, when my daughter could die?!'

"Knowing that all of us were all holding hands 'virtually' around the world giving each other strength, guidance and support on the internet gave me so much courage and strength to face the illness and eventually bring my daughter back to full health."

Finally, Gina said: "It's hard to know exactly how things would have been different without the internet as it's such an integral part of our lives these days. But for me it's summed up by two things: information and community. I guess in the bad old days of no internet, I could have gone to the library to do research and find books, but what the internet gave me was virtually instant access to information - what books to buy, what websites to look at, what research to read, etc. And then I found others like me! On the wonderful ATDT forum I found people going through the same thing I was going through, and they were always there, always willing to share advice, to offer support and a shoulder to cry on. Without that community I would have felt so alone.

"Without the internet I may not have known what the most recent evidence-based research was saying. I may not have known that there were alternatives to the kind of treatment we were getting and learn what was working for other people - and I may not have found new friends all over the world who understood exactly the nightmare I was living through."

By the same author

"Please Eat... A Mother's Struggle To Free Her Teenage Son From Anorexia" by Bev Mattocks

"I have just finished *Please Eat...* and it such a powerful page turner! Bev Mattocks has captured the complexity of her family's journey so honestly, bravely and with such clarity of writing. It is a compelling read." - *Susan Ringwood, Chief Executive, Beat*

"*Please Eat...* is an essential read for anyone trying to understand more about eating disorders in teenage boys. Bev Mattocks describes the story of her son's anorexia but also provides insight for other families facing this complex illness in a world where anorexia is still associated with teenage girls. Totally recommended." - *Sam Thomas, Founder of Men Get Eating Disorders Too*

"I've been reading *Please Eat...* and found it very moving and well written. It was gripping and very insightful. I think people will gain much in terms of strategies, too. It's a really helpful book and we will be recommending it to all our callers with boys. We will also be featuring it on our new website." - *Jane Smith, Director, ABC (Anorexia & Bulimia Care)*

"Cancel your plans for the day when you open this book." - *Laura Collins, Founder of F.E.A.S.T. & Author of Eating With Your Anorexic*

"This is a wonderful book. It's quite hard to read because the story is so painful, but easy to read because of the clarity and simplicity of style." - *Gill Todd, RMN MSc, former Clinical Nurse Leader at the Gerald Russell Eating Disorders Unit, Bethlem & Maudsley Hospitals, London*

"The world is slowly coming to realise that 'Boys Get Anorexia Too'. Bev Mattocks writes honestly and from the heart about helping her teenage son to overcome anorexia. Like ours, this is another success story of a family working together with friends, school and clinicians to beat this insidious illness. Many families will find great comfort from reading this story as well as much needed energy to fight the eating disorder." - *Jenny Langley, Author of Boys Get Anorexia Too*

"Bev Mattocks shares her painful personal story so beautifully that the reader feels a deep connection. She models the tenacity needed by parents to stand up to these deadly illnesses for the long haul. This is a powerful account which health care providers around the world need to read before meeting with their first eating disorders patient." - *Becky Henry, Founder of the Hope Network, LLC & Award Winning Author of Just Tell Her To Stop: Family Stories of Eating Disorders*

"*Please Eat...* is gut wrenching and touching. It captivated me and I could hardly breathe as I was reading it. I read the first six chapters in one sitting. Bev Mattocks has done such a great job of bringing her story to us in a vivid and personal way." - *Parent*

"Bev Mattocks is doing such amazing work empowering other parents and helping to raise awareness that boys get eating disorders too." - *Leah Dean, Executive Director, F.E.A.S.T.*

"This book takes you on an emotional journey through the everyday reality of dealing with anorexia. If you're a health professional, read it to understand what parents are struggling with at home. If your friends or relatives think that anorexia is simply a refusal to eat, get them to read Ben's story. And if you believe anorexia is a girl thing, this book will sweep away your misconceptions." - *Eva Musby, Parent and Writer*

"I have just finished *Please eat...* It is brilliant, well written, evocative and inspirational. I will definitely recommend it to anyone I come across who has a child with an eating disorder." *Caroline, Social Worker, Manchester*

"When I first came across Bev Mattocks' story I was in the depths of despair with my daughter's anorexia which was spiralling out of control. Bev helped me realise that we were not alone, that we could help our daughter to recover and that, as her parents, we were part of solution and not the cause of her eating disorder. This is an empowering book." - *Parent*

"Professionals have written general descriptions from the dry and medical to the flowery and fanciful, but I have never read a better book for describing what it is REALLY like to watch helplessly as a loved one is taken over by the beast that is an eating disorder." - *Parent*

"From page 1, the struggle, the journey, the fight, the ups and downs; becoming Indiana Jones striding through the unpredictability of what the 'demon' (anorexia) will do next but winning in the end. Heart-warming, gut-wrenching; with a wonderful ending of the 'light at the end of a long tunnel' variety and knowing recovery is 100% achievable, but not in a straight line." - *Parent*

"This book is a 'must read' on so many levels. It is well written, compelling, informative and inspirational. Best of all, it's encouraging that a full recovery is possible." - *Parent*

"Please Eat... A Mother's Struggle To Free Her Teenage Son From Anorexia" by Bev Mattocks is available from Amazon and as a Kindle download

Acknowledgements

I am immensely grateful to all the families that willingly and enthusiastically agreed to talk to me for this book. Some I have known for a few years, though the F.E.A.S.T. network, and others are families who I've come to know through the writing of this book.

All of you are truly awesome and I admire you greatly. Sharing your highly personal stories takes courage and I am aware that every single one of you has done this because you care about other families who are facing this dreadful illness. You are also keen to raise awareness of exactly what life is like on the "front line", in the home, outside the cosy confines of the consulting room.

A huge thank you to the young people themselves for demonstrating the courage, grit and determination to fight this illness and win. You are all amazing and I wish you the very best for a wonderful future.

Thank you to Professor Janet Treasure OBE PhD FRCP FRCPsych for writing the *Foreword* and to Laura Collins, founder of F.E.A.S.T. for... well... founding F.E.A.S.T. Virtually every family in this book says that it was a lifeline and a source of knowledge and support that was - and still is - second to none. Thank you, Laura, for offering to write the *Introduction*. Thank you to Becky Henry, Founder of the Hope Network, LLC & Award Winning Author of *Just Tell Her To Stop: Family Stories Of Eating Disorders* for offering advice during initial planning for this book and for writing the *Preface*.

Thank you to the healthcare professionals that spared the time to talk to me: my local GP, the RCGP, Becky Hibbs of the Eating Disorders Unit at the Institute of Psychiatry, King's College London, and Ursula Philpot (Senior Lecturer at Leeds Metropolitan University's School of Health & Wellbeing, Advanced Practice Dietician and Mental Health Group Education Officer for the British Dietetic Association) to name but a few.

Thank you to all the other people I have met in my four-year journey into the complex world of eating disorders - families across the globe that have all shown an interest in this book and my other book: *Please Eat...* and others who follow my blog: *Anorexiaboyrecovery.*

Although I have only met a handful of you in the flesh, I feel as if we are the best of friends. If you can bear the thought of dragging yourself up to Yorkshire at any time, you are most welcome to pop in for a cup of Yorkshire tea!

Resources

Websites

www.aroundthedinnertable.org - The *Around The Dinner Table* forum provides support for parents and caregivers of anorexia, bulimia and other eating disorder patients

www.FEAST-ed.org - *F.E.A.S.T. (Families Empowered And Supporting Treatment of Eating Disorders)* is an international organisation of, and for, parents to help loved ones recover from eating disorders by providing information and mutual support, promoting evidence-based treatment, and advocating for research and education

www.b-eat.co.uk - *Beat* provides helplines, online support and a network of UK-wide self-help groups to help adults and young people in the UK beat their eating disorders

www.mengetedstoo.co.uk - *Men Get Eating Disorders Too* is a UK based charity dedicated to representing and supporting the needs of men with eating disorders

www.maudsleyparents.org - *Maudsley Parents* is a US based volunteer organisation of parents who have helped their children recover from anorexia and bulimia through the use of a Family-Based Treatment known as the Maudsley Approach

www.anorexiabulimiacare.org.uk - *ABC* is a UK national eating disorder organisation that supports sufferers, their families and friends towards full recovery from eating disorders

www.thenewmaudsleyapproach.co.uk - A resource for professionals and carers of people with eating disorders

www.kartiniclinic.com - the *Kartini Clinic* is a US based medical and mental health treatment facility dedicated exclusively to the treatment of eating disorders in children and young adults - this website includes useful information, videos, etc

www.drsarahravin.com - *Dr Sarah Ravin* is a US based eating disorders therapist whose website includes a highly informative blog plus other useful information

www.anorexiaboy.co.uk - my website which talks about our fight to help our son recover from anorexia

www.youtube.com/user/CandMedPRODUCTIONS/videos - C&M Productions is an eating disorder resource for carers promoting evidenced-based treatment and hope in video format

http://eatingdisorders.ucsd.edu – the *University of California, San Diego, Eating Disorders Center for Treatment and Research*

www.youthhealthtalk.org/young_people_Eating_disorders - a project by the *Health Experiences Research Group at the University of Oxford* where young people talk about their experiences of living with, and recovering from, an eating disorder

www.youngminds.org.uk - *Young Minds* is the UK's leading charity committed to improving the emotional wellbeing and mental health of children and young people

Books

Please Eat... A Mother's Struggle To Free Her Teenage Son From Anorexia - by Bev Mattocks

Skills-Based Learning For Caring For A Loved One With An Eating Disorder: The New Maudsley Method - by Janet Treasure

Help Your Teenager Beat an Eating Disorder - by David Lock & Daniel Le Grange

Treating Bulimia In Adolescents: A Family-Based Approach - by David Lock & Daniel Le Grange

Decoding Anorexia: How Breakthroughs In Science Offer Hope For Eating Disorders - by Carrie Arnold

A Collaborative Approach To Eating Disorders – edited by June Alexander and Janet Treasure

Brave Girl Eating: The Inspirational True Story Of One Family's Battle With Anorexia - by Harriet Brown

Just Tell Her To Stop: Family Stories Of Eating Disorders - by Becky Henry, Founder of the Hope Network, LLC

Eating With Your Anorexic - by Laura Collins

Running on Empty: A Diary of Anorexia and Recovery - by Carrie Arnold

A Girl Called Tim: Escape from an Eating Disorder Hell - by June Alexander

Boys Get Anorexia Too - by Jenny Langley

Hope With Eating Disorders: A Self-Help Guide For Parents, Carers And Friends Of Sufferers - by Lynn Crilly

My Kid Is Back: Empowering Parents to Beat Anorexia Nervosa - by June Alexander

Blogs

anorexiaboyrecovery.blogspot.co.uk - my blog

ed-bites.blogspot.co.uk - a blog by Carrie Arnold, author and recovered former anorexia sufferer

www.laurassoapbox.net - a blog by Laura Collins, founder of F.E.A.S.T. and ATDT

charlotteschuntering.blogspot.co.uk - a blog by Charlotte, one of the ATDT members

http://hopenetwork.info/beckys-blog - a blog by Becky Henry, Founder of the Hope Network, LLC

http://www.blog.drsarahravin.com - a blog by Dr Sarah Ravin

Printed in Great Britain
by Amazon.co.uk, Ltd.,
Marston Gate.